HEALTHY LIVING

through

"Dosha Healing"

HEALTHY LIVING

through

"Dosha Healing"

AYURVEDA

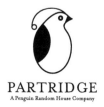

PARTRIDGE

A Penguin Random House Company

ISBN: Hardcover   978-1-4828-2105-5
         Softcover   978-1-4828-2104-8
         eBook   978-1-4828-2103-1

To order additional copies of this book, contact
Partridge India
000 800 10062 62
orders.india@partridgepublishing.com

www.partridgepublishing.com/india

CONTENTS

DEDICATION

I dedicate my book to my soul-mate, *Alok Krishan*, who has always been my Friend, Philosopher & Guide with the trust that I can heal many through spreading the virtues of ancient wisdom of healing.

FOREWORD

I am of the firm belief that each one of us is a by-product of myriad experiences gathered over life times. Thus we have karma, accumulated store house of experiences and desires garnered from one's own karmic journey and also distilled into us by our forefathers DNA and their journeys, and of course our immediate family, especially grand-parents and parents and then, one has home environment, upbringing, school, peers, diet and the environment that each one is brought up in and exposed to . . . . all of this and most importantly one's own individuality . . . . that ascertains one's mental, emotional, physical and spiritual break up and eventually how each individual puzzle fits into the larger composite scheme of things; making you who you are, or at least what you think of yourself and the image you give of yourself to others. Whew! Fabulously and confusingly simple!

In my journey as an author, film maker, journalist and mainly as a counsellor or a spiritual quack, if you may, I have met scores of people who have divulged or often, who have been shown the mirror and thus realized that there are certain attributes about them that they have no real control. I have my fair share of weaknesses, be it physical, emotional, intellectual or spiritual, and I have often tried to overcome them or keep them at bay, but the cards have been dealt with and I have no other option but to play the game the best way I can, but with the cards that aren't going to change.

Take for example, why are some of us, born to the same parents, born and brought up in the same environment and given the same diet and opportunities and virtually are so diverse in nature and the way the body and mind, deals with various issues, including health and wellness? Twin brothers who are as similar as chalk and cheese? Why?

That is why I enjoyed Dr Sonica Krishan's Healthy Living through Dosha Healing. Sonica is an author, speaker, health writer, columnist, editor, Ayurveda consultant and holistic healing coach in the areas of healthy and joyous living through Ayurveda, meditation, yoga and other contemplative practices. The ideal person to help us understand ourselves, then find out our strengths, weaknesses, limitations, and then be able to help our physical, emotional, mental and spiritual growth, by knowing what we can bank on, what needs changes, and what might be difficult to change. Once we have our road map, reaching our destination becomes easier.

Our sages, thousands of years ago, understood the diversity and yet uniformity in creation. They researched and realized that there was a method in the madness, where nature's creation was concerned. They have left very beautiful, clear foot prints, in the sand of time and Dr Sonica Krishan, has to her credit, done them proud.

Ruzbeh N Bharucha
Author, Editor and Documentary Filmmaker

ACKNOWLEDGEMENTS

This book is a sequel to my previously published book '*Healing through Ayurveda*'. Completing this book has been like a dream come true. Ever since I could relate to and appreciate the play of Dosha Healing in the day-to-day living, I have cherished this vision to bring forward Ayurveda's ancient wisdom to the world. But nurturing the dream and making it to happen called for much conviction in my work. I want to thank my mom, Smt. Meera Sharma, who has offered unwavering support for my project. I am also grateful to my kids, Ishita and Ishan, and my entire family as they helped me put in much of time and concentration that writing a book demands. Earnest thanks to Ruzbeh Barucha for the beautiful foreword and also for encouraging me to come up in story telling manner with the ancient concept. Thank you Shiv Joshi for putting in effort in editing the book for me.

Special thanks and heart felt gratitude to my colleagues, seniors and prominent authors who are masters in their arena—Roxana Jones, Dr. Marc Halpern, Catherine Fenske, Jane Scarratt, Dr Talavane Krishna, Debbie Friend, Anton Van Den Berg, Dr Amit Nagpal, Tanya Markul, Rory Kelly Connor, Carly Alyssa Thorne and Linda Lycett, Philippe Matthews for their exceptional effort and kind gesture to have endorsed my book in the most candid words.

Also, I am always grateful to my dear readers and all those who have keen interest and faith in keeping the 5000 years old Ayurveda healing alive through their practice, reading, writing, speaking and also teaching. It is surely the true dedication that provides with great inspiration to spread the light and wisdom that the science of Ayurveda bestows.

INTRODUCTION

What's this Book About?

This is a story about three friends, whose lives changed drastically due a fourth someone. But the change was total. They grew up together as little girls and the threesome was inseparable. They played together, stayed together and studied together. They were with each other through the highs and lows of entire childhood, which cemented their bond. That's why even after they grew up and as it happens to all of us—had to go their separate ways—they kept in touch and were still close to each other's heart. Unlike a lot of 'best friends' of childhood, the three managed to keep the glow of friendship alive.

However, when their paths crossed once again something happened. A fourth someone—*Dr Ayur Wizard*—came along and turned their lives upside down, albeit in a virtuous way. He went on to become a friend, philosopher and guide to the three. It was he who helped educate the three friends (and the readers) about the 'whats' and the 'whys', the pros and the cons of all that concerns health, wisdom and happiness. But let's not get ahead of ourselves here. Let's stick to talking about the girls because it is through knowing the girls that you will learn about fundamentals of health as per Ayurveda.

PROLOGUE

CHAPTER 1

The Terrific Three

Childhood friends, as they are often referred to jokingly, Vani, Pia and Kavya, lived a few houses away from each other in a bustling neighbourhood of Delhi. Pia and Kavya knew each other and their families since the time the girls started knowing themselves. Vani joined the gang much later, in class two, when her father came to the city, on transfer. She hit it off instantly with the other two and since then they were thick as thieves till life happened and took them away from each other to three different cities.

Vani pursued a career in IT and landed a job as a software professional at the IT hub of Bengaluru. So immersed was she in her work that she didn't find the time to even look for an eligible spouse. As the years flew by, she came to the conclusion that perhaps marriage was not her cup of tea. It was then that Harshit came and swept her off her feet. She had finally found her life partner, who, incidentally also was from the same industry as hers.

Pia took up hotel management and later settled into a live-in relationship with Rahul, her nine years senior. Rahul wasn't so much the man of her dreams, but he seemed to be the best one out there, and Pia knew she could always rely on him. More importantly, he could live with Pia's short temper and the tantrums she threw. She was comfortable in their arrangement together, which was based more on convenience than compatibility. Moreover, it was minus the constraints of a marital relationship, and the baggage of futile expectations that comes with it.

In the meanwhile, Kavya, who usually was just happy doing nothing, had landed herself a government job. She was the Information and Communication representative with the Information and Broadcasting department with Indian Government. She loved her job, her life and more than everything, Aarnav, her doctor husband. In her free time, she would spend some time at his clinic, making herself useful doing small chores. She didn't know why but while she was there she felt so much at home with his patients.

The three friends are now in their late thirties and after nine long years of separation, have decided to meet again at the very place that had brought them together so many years back: their parents' home, back in good old Delhi. Where else?

Getting to know them better

Thanks to her slim and tall figure, **Vani** had always been the envy of her friends and foes alike. Whatever the girl ate just never showed! As if to rub it in, she emphasised her lean silhouette by choosing markedly short dresses. Still she wasn't all pleased about her looks. Her grouse: the dark complexion. It worried her a lot, especially before finding a groom. But her husband seemed to have accepted her and had even playfully given her the nickname *Saloni*. That wasn't all; she had more hidden fears. And they were with her ever since she actualised the concept of beauty during her mid-teens.

Vani had noticed then that not only her complexion was on the darker side; but her skin also was rough. At such a tender age, she quietly emptied bottles of crèmes and body lotions to camouflage the aridness and demonstrate a smooth texture. Her mother kept telling her to always apply coconut oil on her damp body just after bath so as to restore the moisture. But Vani was too overwhelmed with herself to pay much heed.

Now, over the years, her skin showed early signs of ageing: she already had wrinkles and sparing hair. Why? This question lingered at the back of her mind, almost constantly. Nevertheless, she was a keen follower of all the latest anti-ageing beauty drama. If it was the latest, she would go for. It didn't matter to her that the fad hardly authenticated much response. She knew that she just couldn't stick to one therapy or beauty treatment for long.

The hassles of daily life, undue stress, work and home pressure and her age gap with her kid, were all robbing her of her splendour. Her latest anxiety was early baldness: her hair was so brittle all the while. But fearing that he could not understand, she didn't breathe a word about it to her husband. Even if he did understand, Vani just didn't want to suffer his sermons about diet improvement and health management! She'd rather fret. Although she would never admit, she silently admired Harshit's glowing skin and cool attitude and wondered how he could be so different!

Pia was blessed with a fair and glowing complexion. But since early teenage years, she had fought a losing battle with acne and freckles. Actually, she had oily skin which got greasier every now and then. Long back her doctor had advised her to stay clear of spicy and fried foods: it was the advice she had followed religiously.

But the girl wasn't the kind to be overtly bothered with looks, ever. She wasn't the careless type, but there was so much more in the world to strain the nerves. Besides, she hadn't much to worry about either. She was neither thin nor obese, though she tended to gain a few pounds. Since she was aware of this, Pia just wouldn't let sluggishness set in. But she also knew that she couldn't stick to regimes for long—not because of lack of will power, but because her stamina would just give out. Once on a diet regime, she could be disciplined with herself. Even the gruelling gym sessions could not dampen her enthusiasm. However, eventually, she would feel totally drained. This had happened many times now. So she was more particular about not putting on weight and then deplete out the time, money and energy just to regain fitness. Yes, Pia was an incorrigible fitness freak. She would go through health journals, diet plans and lay out meal regimes for the entire family. No matter what, she followed it all. Although, being unlike her, others in her family could not continue the same for long. And this agonised and irritated the girl to no end.

However, despite all this, she looked fit and was admired for her now glowing and wrinkle free skin. Besides the acne in her teens, beauty wise she had never any problem. Though not the prettiest girl in town, she was fit and, for Pia, this was more important. Now, at her age, there were a few greys, which made her livid at times. So she had taken to visiting saloons more frequently to get her hair synthetically coloured.

Kavya had always been chubby. Perhaps it was due to the high fat milk she feasted on as a child. When she was a little kid, her family had kept a buffalo at home, which was milked every day. So she indulged in the high fat milk, crèmes and homemade lumps of white butter that her granny would allow her to delight in. Another explanation Kavya gave herself was her sweet tooth: she just couldn't resist sweets.

Sweets, ice creams, cakes and chocolates were temptations she just couldn't evade. More than delicacies, they were mood boosters, her emotional respites. The sweets helped soothe her troubles and she felt all was well when she had them. Kavya knew that constantly eating foods high in sugar added to her weight. But it didn't matter to her. Convinced, that the healthy frame represented robustness, she often turned a deaf ear to the comments her slim doctor husband Aarnav passed on her weightiness. When together, the couple did seem physical opposites of each other. But instead of feeling bad for not watching her weight, Kavya used to get angry at Aarnav for not putting on weight instead.

Apart from her weight, Kavya was okay with her skin texture, which felt soft and supple. Her complexion too was reasonably fair, though her skin always felt cool. Her hair was black, thick and wavy. On the whole, she felt she looked quite good. In fact, she even felt proud for defying all the early signs of aging even at 39.

If only she were a little slim, she would look so much more attractive and younger! But, Kavya didn't mind it all that much. Or so it seemed. For, now, in her late thirties, she had started feeling frequently worn out. And though she wouldn't admit it to anyone, it kept her all the more lethargic and exhausted.

CHAPTER 2

And They Meet Again!

Now that you know a little bit about the three, let's get back to our story where the three friends decide to meet after a long gap of nine years. A lot of co-ordination on WhatsApp and other social networking sites later, finally the day arrived when the three met at their old neighbourhood in Delhi. When they actually met, as was expected, they created quite a racket, yelling and squealing like little girls. They were literally jumping up and down. Mixed with laughter came the tears unbidden—happy tears, all around.

"Feels so good to see you! It feels just like it did before we were all married," said Pia, between sobs.

"Ya, just imagine we are here. All three of us, together once again like before, without the hassles of running after the kids or bearing with our hubbies," said Vani, winking.

This was her very first time she was on holiday alone, leaving her daughter and husband behind and she was strangely feeling happy about it.

"I'm happy to see you girls, but I don't think it will be really different from our daily lives," muttered a cheerless Kavya. Vani and Pia looked at each other and shrugged, as if to say, 'what's with her?' They were both aware that their friend had changed and was no longer the bubbly jovial person that she always was.

"Oh come on, Kavya. Now that all three of us are together, we're going to rule the world, just like we did in the good old days," Vani attempted to cheer up her friend. Then she got up and hugged Kavya tight, not letting go till she squeezed a smile out of her friend.

"Friends! Friends!" shouted Pia, clapping to get everybody's attention.

"Listen, in addition to the usual fun stuff, this time, let's do something different—something that will be good for all of us. Mom told me about some special classes being held in town. It seems the guy provides advice on dietary and lifestyle modifications based on some ancient Indian science."

"Count me out of this," grumbled Kavya. "I am done with Babas, healers and their ilk. They claim to relieve you of your problems, transform your life . . . . blah, blah, blah . . . . but all they do is end up relieving you of your money," she scoffed.

"So true! Why waste our resources on a guy who is anyway going to tell us what we already know? Instead, let's just freak out and relax during our privileged vacation!" Vani joined in.

"How do you know what he'll say? From what mom tells me, this fellow sounds like the real deal. Lots of people have benefitted from following his advice. We'll have fun, but there's no chance I'm going to miss out on this 'talk of the town' health counselling," declared Pia, always the die-hard health freak. "Besides, Ayurveda is 'in'," she added.

"Oh puhleez! I don't see anything new to learn from this primeval pathy. Remember, we have virtually grown up with taking Chavanprash and decoctions like that. What good did that do to us?" countered Vani. "Moreover, the philosophy is meant to impress only the poor and uneducated," she added without a pause.

"Did you just say Ayurveda?" asked Kavya turning to Pia. "Why didn't you first say it was Ayurveda?" she demanded. "Like it would have made a difference," said Pia, rolling her eyes.

"Helloo, I have some knowledge of Ayurveda. If you remember, my husband is a doctor and I've accompanied him on seminars abroad. Did you know how much foreigners respect Ayurveda? I was so proud to find so many doctors eager to learn about our inherent ancient therapeutic science," said Kavya emphatically.

"Just a few minutes back, you were totally against it. Now, it's a science?" asked an incredulous Vani.

"I call it science because I have had the chance to understand the philosophies. And tell you what, they have utterly impressed me," asserted Kavya.

"Really?" asked Vani, now clearly baffled by the sudden change in Kavya's attitude at the mere mention of Ayurveda.

'Yes, I have a mountain of literature on this ancient science and its efficacy. If you want, I can mail you the stuff," Kavya offered.

"If you have all the literature and have attended so many seminars, tell me how come you're still fat?," spat Vani, feeling bitter for having lost the battle now that Kavya too had changed sides.

She regretted it the instance the words left her mouth. But the damage had been done and Kavya was in tears. "I'm so sorry, I'm so sorry . . . my friend, I didn't mean it. Please forgive me," pleaded Vani, who was now feeling like shit for having hurt her friend's feelings.

"If you really feel sorry from the bottom of your heart, show it by joining us for the counselling session on Ayurveda," said Pia with a wink.

And the three burst out laughing.

Chapter 3

Meet Dr Ayur Wizard

Finally, the girls decided to give the Ayurveda guy a chance. They would attend just one session and as Vani had warned, "If we don't like it, we're not going to go back, no matter what."

So the next morning, not knowing what to expect, the girls parked themselves in the room, which was surprisingly full.

"Thank God, there's quite a crowd. We are not the only suckers," joked Vani.

Just then the murmur in the class died down as Dr Ayur Wizard walked in. Tall and confident, the Wizard was somewhere between 40 to 50 years old. The glow on his face, his posture and his visibly fit body, made it difficult to put an exact number on his age. To top it, he was quite good looking and had a charming smile, which he was now beaming, full throttle at his crowd.

"Oh, he's so cute. If nothing, at least, I can feast my eyes," whispered Vani to the others. "Shh . . . said Kavya," elbowing her.

"Good Morning," said Dr Wizard in a voice that was at once authoritative and soothing. "I will speak to people in batches as it's a counselling session," he said. With that he divided the audience into groups and the first group turned out to be Vani, Pia and Kavya.

Once the others left, Dr Wizard addressed the three, "Today, I will introduce you to the ancient wisdom of Ayurveda and specifically to the concept of Dosha healing. Let me tell you that the word Ayurveda evokes interest and scepticism in equal measures. There is a lot said, heard and written about it. And while a lot of it might be true, there are things that aren't. People have intrigue about it as well as qualms and I will first clear the air before we proceed any further," said Dr Wizard sweeping his gaze at the three.

"I can see the stupefied look on your lovely faces already, but please lend me an ear for the next five minutes and I promise you that these five minutes will be a crucial time in your life—it might well be the time that will work like an anchor for your physical, mental and spiritual health," he proclaimed.

"Mark my words ladies, an anchor!' he repeated, raising his brows.

He now had their full attention. "What if I tell you that understanding Dosha Healing is going to be a great aid in losing weight?" he asked, staring straight into Kavya's eyes. Kavya was stunned. His words struck a nerve, and her eyes welled up.

"What's more, what if I tell you that this will also help you get rid of whatever physical and mental afflictions you are facing at this age?" he continued, walking towards her. He came up to her and before she could reply, patted her shoulder conveying that he understood her predicament. That broke the dam and tears streamed down Kavya's face. But these weren't tears of sadness, but of relief. At last, someone had understood how she felt.

He then turned to Vani. "What if I assure you that your session with me would help you acquire your mental balance and tranquillity? And not to forget your dreams of getting fairly glowing, smooth skin and freedom from tension headaches. Sounds good?" That did the trick for Vani, who was beaming like a beacon. All reservations about attending the class fled her mind. She was already imagining herself as the new confident, striking woman, alluring the world with her charisma.

Surprisingly, it was Pia who played the devil's advocate. "But how do you intend to guarantee that we are going to accomplish all that you swear by?" she demanded.

"Hold it right there," he shot back. "Neither I am swearing by anything, nor am I claiming some sort of miracle cures, young lady," said the man.

"And let me remind you, my five minutes are not over yet; there are still two minutes to go," he reminded.

"All I can say with conviction is that your gains could be bountiful in terms of having articulate and pleased mental frame, and you could relieve yourself from the discrepancy of being impatient and heated so easily," he said with a knowing smile.

"Let me make you understand it with a different approach. You're pursuing your career in hotel management, right?"

'So, this guy has already enquired about us?' Pia mused to herself.

"Now, don't be surprised. I read it in the form you filled," he said as if reading her mind.

"Now, tell me this: while preparing different recipes, how often do you use the same ingredients in your cooking?"

"Oh come on," said Pia. "If I use the same stuff over and over again in all dishes, the food will turn out to be so boooring".

"That's exactly my point. It's the same with us humans, you and me. If we all follow the same health rules, it's of

33

no use. In fact, we could be doing ourselves more harm than good," he said.

"It's hardly a good analogy . . . recipes and humans," Pia pointed out. "Right, but it helped make the point that same rules of health don't apply to all. Simply because we are all not the same, just like all recipes are not the same," he said.

"Pia, if I tell you to include sweet in your diet more often to help you keep fit and also acquire psychological gains, will you do this?"

Pia answered with a nod.

"But Kavya, if you follow the same diet advice I just gave your friend, in your case, it will lead to just the opposite. Vani, what if I told you sleeping early at night, coupled with an oil massage to the soles of your feet could leave you much relaxed and affirmative, does this sound reassuring to you?"

Vani just stared back in amazement, thinking, 'Who the hell was this guy. Some sort of astrologer or what?'

Just then Dr Wizard looked at his watch and said, "And this concludes our five minutes session. Young ladies, now the ball is in your court. Please go out, breathe in some fresh air, take your time to discuss with each other and then come back in and tell me if you want to continue with me. If you return by end of the day, I'll take that as a yes. If you don't, I will know your answer. Good luck".

A little dazed, the girls filed out of the room in silence. Once out, they all just looked at each other, waiting for someone to break the spell. Now the big question was: will they return to Dr Wizard?

CHAPTER 4

Introduction to The Three Steps

Well, you guessed right. The girls went back, and soon. And this time, none of them had to persuade the other to return; the decision was unanimous. They all wanted to benefit from Dosha Healing.

As if expecting them Dr Wizard sat unperturbed and continued as if nothing had happened. "Now that you've decided to try Dosha Healing, the guide to transformation using Ayurveda Lifestyle, let me make one thing clear right at start. I'm not here to give you some medicine prescriptions or teach you how to perform ancient deep breathing techniques of Pranayama. I am also not going ask you about your diseases or present an analysis of your afflictions. And don't expect me to conduct some sort of a lecture about Ayurveda . . ."

"Then what are we here for?" interrupted Pia, with a frown. "I was responsible for bringing my friends here. And I thought this would be some kind of lifestyle counselling with positive overtones for the three of us and our families. But from what you say, it feels like it's going to be a waste of our time, money and energy" she complained.

"I agree with Pia" Vani joined in.

"I think we better get a refund. I was actually not convinced right from the time I heard about your class, but my friends are the only reason I am here. Besides, Kavya has been gaining weight uncontrollably and has been facing health doldrums. And I was secretly hoping for her sake that you may have some ancient cure or herb remedy that could help her. Right Kavya?" Pia turned towards her friend only to find her staring into the unknown and with a complete blank look on her face.

'Ok ladies, I understand what you mean. But be honest and tell me how long did you have to wait to get an appointment with me?" The girls kept quiet, their silence revealing their answer. Fact was, since they decided, they had to make several calls and still had been put on a waiting list. It was only in the last week of their vacation that finally they could get through. Getting an appointment with Dr Wizard hadn't exactly been cakewalk. It was true that people were benefitting from Dr Wizard's approach. They got their answer.

"I didn't mean to offend you. But I will just say one thing that this is going to be a life changing experience for you all. But since you still have doubts, I will ask you to reconsider."

Just when Pia was about to say something, Kavya cut in, "We are here to learn from you and I would request each one here to be enduring and let the workshop commence." She sounded determined. Her friends, now tight-lipped, only nodded their consent.

'Fine. Let us begin our journey with Dosha Healing—The Ayurveda Lifestyle transformation guide and here's the pathway we are going to take," he said turning to write something on a white board.

This is what he wrote:

Step One: Self-Identification

Step Two: Self-Understanding

Step Three: Self-Management

'That's all?' Vani asked astounded.

"Yes, that is all. Believe it or not, at the end of Step Three, all three of you are going to emerge transformed. You will be winners. By the virtue of what Ayurveda will teach you, you are going to succeed in the race of gaining 'natural' wellbeing," said Ayur wizard, stressing on the word 'natural'.

"Tomorrow, we begin with step 1. You have to first understand your own basic nature. So that you are able to impede all the allegations whatsoever you could consciously or subconsciously be aiming at your own self. So, my very first direction to you, till we begin tomorrow is this: Stop being a target of your own accusation."

Once again, the girls were stunned into silence.

Chapter 5

Step One: Self-Identification

The next day, which was the first class of Dosha healing session, the three friends were now to acknowledge the very first step of Self-Identification. Not knowing what to expect and with a bit of apprehension about what exactly 'understanding your basic nature' meant, the three friends sat in Dr Wizard's class. When he came in, he picked up a look of scepticism on their faces as well. Greeting them with a knowing smile, he began, "Good Morning Ladies. Let's begin by each one of you telling me about your experiences as a mother you are."

'Huh? Where did this come from,' thought Vani, who was half expecting him to ask about her personal preferences or even health issues.

Recovering quickly, she mumbled, as if thinking out loud, "Mmm . . . . let me think. I believe I'm like any other mom . . . in the sense that like everyone else, I worry all the time when my child is not besides me. I am generally concerned and anxious and keep feeling that something wrong is going to happen to my young one. Don't get me wrong, I've tried not to be over-protective, but as long as my daughter is concerned, I am naturally filled with all sorts of fears and fantasies. Don't we all?" Having never voiced her concerns openly in front of anyone other than her family members, she turned to Pia for validation.

"Well, I do worry at times. But I believe that prevention is better than cure and hence have laid down certain rules and regulations, which I ensure that my 9-year-old son follows. Whether it is his meals, homework, cleanliness or his play sessions, I have chalked out everything. I don't want to be cruel and arrogant all the while, but his age demands that. Luckily, my son is quite an obedient child, but hubby pampers him unnecessarily. Some might say, I'm strict, but I see myself more as a mother who likes discipline," she said with a huff.

"Besides, I feel that when kids near their teens you have to be a little sterner so that they don't stray. And I hate it when my child tries to take me for granted," she said looking pointedly at Kavya, who she felt was too lenient with her children.

Kavya sat unruffled. After a beat, and looking at Dr Wizard she said, "Actually, I have a totally different opinion. I believe in going easy on my cuties. You know, they are young and don't understand stringency. I love my two daughters more than anything in the world. I can never ever think of raising my voice on them. So many times I have had a rift with Aarnav over this. He wants them to be strictly controlled but I want my girls to be kids that they are and enjoy their childhood to the fullest. So, if by any chance, my daughters are scolded or they get hurt, it's me who ends up in tears. But I love to be a protective and cautious mother," she said in earnest. Though, sometimes I do feel like I'm being taken for granted both by my daughters as well as my husband."

"Ok ladies," said Dr Wizard breaking the awkward silence that followed. "So, we have heard about how each one of you plays the role a mother. I started the discussion on this topic on purpose. In my experience, women open up easily even while talking to strangers about their kids. But apart from that, the topic has helped you look at yourself from a third person's point of view and has highlighted the difference in your personalities. Did you notice that although all three of you are mothers, yet you are so different from each other," he said making a mental note of his observation that Vani is an anxious mother, Pia demanding and Kavya is tender. Not that he was judging them, but this was important for what was to follow.

"Understanding yourself and identifying what kind of a person you are is important in Ayurveda," he explained.

"Why's that?" asked Pia.

"Tell me, do we all have same physique and mentality, similar levels of health and stress, identical likes and dislikes or matching needs and tastes for that matter?"

All three shook their head in harmony, just like back in school. When they realised this, they giggled.

Even if he noticed, Dr Wizard didn't show it and continued, "Then how can we derive health and happiness following the same rules of wellness? First thing you need to understand about Ayurveda is that it doesn't believe in one size fits all."

The Ayurveda science of Dosha Healing suggests that there are three basic types of personalities: Vata, Pitta and Kapha. The world we live in is made up of five elements," he said, listing them on the board.

- Aakasha (Sky / Ether)

- Vayu (Air)

- Agni (Fire)

- Jala (Water)

- Prithvi (Earth)

"As in Nature, the same five elements are present within us too. But not in the same proportion. And they are present in the following combinations:

- Ether & Air = Vata Dosha

- Fire = Pitta Dosha

- Earth & Water = Kapha Dosha

So depending on which combination is dominant, each person is either a Vata Type (Ether + Air), Pitta type (Fire) or Kapha type (water + earth). Or, he could be a combination of the three," he explained.

"Isn't it similar to humourism, the Greek propounded several centuries ago? I read it somewhere . . ." asked Kavya.

"Umm . . . . for the sake of comprehending the concept, you may say so. But Ayurveda is a proven science and humourism or humoralism as it was known then was a theory, which is now discredited," he clarified. "Besides humourism believes that we have four fluids in the body. But like I explained, Ayurveda believes that there are five elements present within us. Let's not discuss humourism any further, or you will get confused," Dr Wizard admonished.

To check their understanding, Dr Wizard asked them, "So tell me, which are the main types of personalities according to Ayurveda?"

"Vata Type, which is a combination of ether and air," Kavya offered.

"Pitta type, which means there is only fire element," Pia chimed in.

"Kapha type, which means water and earth," Vani said.

"One could be amalgamation of the three. Or more commonly we find combination personalities with presence of two of the three doshas like Vata-Pitta type, Pitta—Kapha type or Vata—Kapha type," Dr Wizard finished.

"Nevertheless, the three basic types of personalities are Vata type, Pitta type or Kapha type. Each of these types has distinct physical characteristics, looking at which one can identify whether a person is a Vata, Pitta or Kapha," he explained.

"Just by looking at personal physical attributes?" asked a surprised Vani.

"That and by knowing a few personality traits," he replied.

"Here, take these papers, I've listed the attributes on them," he said giving them some documents.

Here's what was written on the paper

You are naturally a 'Vata Type' if you have the following characteristics:

- Tall, skinny and lean.

- Dry and dark skin.

- Early baldness.

- Uncontrollably talkative.

- Walk and eat quickly.

- Jump to conclusions.

- Change decisions often.

Trademark Vata Properties

- Laghu (light): Light boned.

- Ruksha (dry): Dry hair and mouth cavity.

- Shita (cold): Poor circulation.

- Daruna (mobility): Action oriented with erratic digestion.

- Khara (rough): Rough hair and skin

- Vishada (transparency): Mystical approach. The person is a thinker.

You are naturally a 'Pitta type' if you have the following characteristics:

- Yellowish skin, well developed muscles.

- Medium height and proportionate weight.

- Premature greying.

- Intelligent.

- Good stamina, more sweating.

- Easily irritated, judgmental and angry.

Trademark Pitta Properties

- Ushana (hot): Higher than normal body temperature.

- Tikshana (sharp): Sharp memory

- Drava (fluid): Tendency to easy acid formation.

- Sara (mobile): Predisposed to spreading of rashes.

- Snigdha (slightly oily): Smooth, oily skin

You are naturally a 'Kapha type' if you have the following characteristics:

- Whitish skin, smooth hair and nails

- Bulky, with a tendency to be overweight

- Strong, intelligent and calm and composed

- Less talkative

- Stick to decisions

- Slow and steady.

Trademark Kapha Properties

- Guru (heavy): Tendency to gain weight

- Sthira (stable): Sedentary, not easily perturbed

- Snigdha (oily): Soft skin tone and voice

- Pichchila (gelatinous): More than normal saliva, mucous generation.

- Shita (cold): Cool skin

- Shlakshma (smooth): Smooth skin and hair

- Sthula (coarse): Solid bony structure, substantial thoughts.

One of the sheets of papers that he carried, Dr Wizard displayed before them a table to aid self-identification . . . .

Table name: What type are you?

S.No	Physical Features & Mental Temprament	*VATA* (AIR)	*PITTA* (FIRE)	*KAPHA* (PHLEGM)
1.	Body appearance	Thin, lean body	Sensitive and proportionate body.	Full and symmetrical body, tendency of obesity.
2.	Skin color	Blackish	Yellowish or reddish	Fair complexion
3.	Skin appearance	Dry, rough and cracked skin with swollen and visible veins.	Pimples, moles, freckles etc. and reddish lips, ears, hands etc	Slimy, smooth, soft and oily skin
4.	Hair texture	Rough, hard and brittle hair.	Sparse hair growth and premature greying and hair falling	Thick, black and greasy hair, maybe curly
5	Eyes	Dusky and sunken eyes with blackish tinge	Yellow or red coloured	White and lubricous
6	Mouth	Dry	Dry and burning sensation	More production of secretions, phlegm
7	Tongue	Dry, fissured blackish and stained	Reddish colour with black tinge and Ulcerated.	White, moist and coated.

8	Taste	Astringent and distorted	Bitter and sour	Sweet taste in mouth
9	Voice	Cracked and heavy pitch.	Clear speech	Sweet and impressive
10	Thirst	Misleading and unclear	More or excessive	Less
11	Hunger	Hunger pattern and digestion keeps varying	Good digestive power and more hunger.	Less hunger, feeling of fullness after food.
12	Sweat	Less and without smell	More, hot and smelly	Normal and cold
13	Urine	Slightly yellowish with blue tinge	Yellowish and hot, perhaps with red tinge.	Whitish, thick and frothy, somewhat slimy
14	Faeces	Less frequent, constipated, hard, dark and fragile.	Loose, hot, smelly and with burning sensation	Solid and slimy, perhaps with mucous.
15	Nails	Rough, blackish and dry	Reddish or yellowish	White and unctuous
16	Gait	Fast	Normal	Slow
17	Dreams	Flying in the skies	Fire, flame, candles, sun lightening, stars	Sea, rivers, waterfalls, lotus etc
18	Sleep pattern	Less sleep	Less or normal sleep	More sleep, lethargy
20	Nature	Impulsive, Impatient, hasty, hyper, fast, short tempered, indecisive, cowardly.	Hot tempered, irritating, logical, intelligent, witty, brave, clever, ascetic	Sober, patient, humble, stable, tolerant, unexcited, calm and composed, disciplined, lazy and slow

21	Pulse	Zigzag, fast and irregular	Impulsive, heavy and jumping	Smooth, weak and slow
22	Diseases	*Vata Type* 80 diseases	*Pitta Type* 40 diseases	*Kapha Type* 20 diseases
24	Intolerance	Cold	Hot	Cold

"I think we've had enough for the day. What I want you to do is, based on the chart that I've given you, spend some time finding out which of the categories you fall under and complete these self-identification worksheets that now I am giving you," he said, passing around the papers.

"Oh no, home work! We weren't prepared for this. I thought it would only be lectures and presentations. Oh this isn't fair," protested Pia. "You bet! As it is, we're here on vacation, not study. Besides, the vacation too is short? Can we not skip this?" Vani also asked with a snuff. Dr Wizard answered with a question, "This isn't homework it's an exercise. Don't you want to know for yourself what kind of personality you are?" he asked.

That intrigued them enough to drown their protests. "And there's one other thing I want you to do. Don't share your diagnosis with anyone, not even with each other. Because we're going to play a little game. After you've identified your personality, I want you to guess what type your friends are. Let's see how well you know yourself and each other. Good luck!"

CHAPTER 6

The Guessing Game

Once outside, all three started discussing at once. "Well this sucks! I was happy to be away from kid's homework for a few days. And now I'm supposed to do my own homework," Vani grumbled. "I swear!" Pia agreed, literally crushing the exercise sheet that Ayur wizard had forced upon them. "Actually, I don't feel the same way. I'm quite excited to find out whether I am Kapha, Pitta or Vata. But more than that, I'm aching to guess what type you guys are and whether I am right about you," Kavya admitted.

"Well . . . actually, I'm eager too. Only, just don't want this to be boring and takes up too much of my time or makes me ponder over the school days," said Vani. "I'm more interested in finding out how old Dr Ayur Wizard is. He looks so young, and still keeps addressing us as 'young ladies' all the time," she added.

"My thoughts exactly! Even I'm dying to know his age. He's so good looking," Kavya said with a wink. The three giggled together.

"Jokes apart, I think we need to at least go and attempt whatever he has assigned us today. I'm quite impressed by his enthusiasm towards his project. And if he is right even by twenty percent, this means maybe we get what we have come to him for," said an earnest Kavya. The twinkle in her eyes was enough to convince her friends.

"Besides, let's do group study, like we did in the good old days," said Pia, with a mischief in her eyes. "We'll also decide then, whether we want to continue with this workshop. Because I can clearly feel the resistance coming in once again," she said. So they parted deciding to meet again at the coffee shop that evening.

At the decided hour, Vani was the first to reach the Coffee shop. Anxious and yet excited, she started pacing the reception. She finally settled into a chair, when she became mindful of the curious glares of others in the shop. The wait was getting too much for her and she started impatiently tapping the table board with the tips of her fingers. "Hey there, why am I not surprised you showed up first," said Kavya walking in a good 15 minutes late. Yet, she strode like she had all the time in the world. "And why am I not surprised you will come in late," Vani said with sarcasm. "We have more imperative work to do than to sit here waiting for each other," said Kavya teasing Vani, knowing it would further irritate her friend.

"I agree fully," said Pia who joined in. "Jokes apart, I'm really, really fed up of this Delhi traffic. No one has driving sense. Can you believe it? I was in the cab for more than one hour. I feel like suing everybody from the government. How will the country ever make progress like this?" said an obviously angered Pia.

'Pia, Pia calm down. Here, have some water," said Vani calming her friend. "Some things will never change. So let's not waste our breath on them," she said. "Here comes our coffee. I've taken the liberty to order for you guys," she said.

After the coffees arrived, the three friends settled down for coffee and conversation. "Did you guys get a chance to go through the questionnaire? I read it five times and guess what? I am beginning to believe that I am one particular type of personality" said Vani. "Which one?" asked Kavya nibbling at a cookie.

"Hey we're not supposed to reveal, remember?" Vani said.

"Not even to me," asked Kavya making a puppy face.

"Oh hell, now you've had me. I think I'm Vata type," Vani said

"There is so much correspondence both in physical appearance as well as temperament. I'm not 100 percent sure. No, I think I am I'm sure that I am Vata type. Now what do you both have to say on this?" she asked.

"How can you be so sure?" challenged Pia. She had done her home work well and was far more calculative and naturally persuasive among all the three girls. "I think this whole thing is a waste of time" she declared.

"We are all educated and have a modern and logical approach. How can we simply succumb to such primitive studies? It's just some list compiled by God-knows-who," she wondered aloud.

"This sort of self-analysis could be fitting with some people, but it doesn't mean we all fall prey to it and begin to conclude our innate existence. We have no understanding of this, let alone, training. And if for a moment, we believe that we resemble one of the factious personalities as portrayed by the wizard, what is the guarantee that we will get all solutions?" she asked. The others were taken aback by this outburst.

"Well, I at least was in no genuine mood to work out this Self-identification worksheet," said Pia calming down a bit.

"So you haven't done your homework" deduced Vani, sounding perplexed.

"Who said that?" she snapped. "Didn't you just say so yourself?" asked a stupefied Vani.

"I said I was not in the mood. But that doesn't mean I didn't do it. I had to, because Rahul convinced me over the phone," she admitted.

"So, it was Rahul who made you do your self-identification worksheet?' this time Kavya was frowning deliberately sounding cynical.

"He didn't make me do anything. I did it because what he said made sense. He said that I shouldn't disregard what Dr Ayur Wizard could be offering us. Because he did some research on Ayurveda and found that the ancient Indian science is authentic and has helped millions of people. The science is essentially self-explained and relates mainly to how to live our life. It has been, is and always will be the same for mankind. And also that it can't be overlooked," said Pia.

"Now, now look who's talking!" said Vani exasperated.

Kavya was taking it all in, like a silent spectator.

"Rahul made me realise that there's no harm in trying," she said.

"Finally, some sense," said Vani.

"So, at least, I went through the set of questions" said Pia.

"And you've found that you are a Pitta personality?" this came from Kavya, who finally broke her silence.

Pia nodded.

"What about you?" Vani asked Kavya, who seemed eager to share her guess with her friends.

"I am Kapha type. Actually, I had suspected this all along and the 90-95 per cent scoring I got in the self-identity questionnaire confirmed it. Knowing that whatever I am—my physique, basic nature, preferences is natural—brought in a kind of peace."

"The Kapha type of person is naturally slow and steady" Kavya continued. "So, people like me are calm and composed. They are also 'naturally' sweet-toothed and this explains my craving for sweets, chocolates and ice-creams," she said, almost salivating imagining her favourite foods.

"So, you are clear about your personality and therefore would be patiently waiting for tomorrow's class?" queried Pia.

"Not really" said Kavya, sounding confused for the first time. "I am so convinced that I am naturally a Kapha person. This has helped me accept myself with all the good and the bad, because that's who I am naturally. Now, I'm really not sure whether I need to go through the tedious healing sessions with Dr Ayur Wizard," she said.

"I think you have a point there," said Vani. "Let's assume that you are right about you being Kapha type and Pia being Pitta type. And let's say I am Vata type. If we are naturally meant to be the way we are, what help can we expect in this case?" she wondered. "I mean, what healing could he have to offer us if God has made us so?"

"True. But don't you think there's all the more reason we should go and find out? Let's just attend tomorrow's class and see how it goes. We have our goods and we have our bads, as per his hypothesis. So now let's see how he plans to help us. If we find that this guy is trying to play with our sentiments, then we'll give it to him," said Pia banging her fist on the coffee table. Once again, it was decided that they would give Dr Wizard another chance.

CHAPTER 7

Finding the Answers

"Welcome back ladies. I assume you all have done your homework," Dr Ayur Wizard said with a smile. His gaze swept across the three faces. "And I'm sure, being the kind of friends you are, you have discussed this amongst yourselves," he surmised, surprising them all. "And that's ok."

"So instead of you telling me about what you have guessed, let me start by expressing your types and you can check if you've deduced correctly," he said.

'Now, Vani you are a Vata type . . . in fact a typical Vata personality," he said looking straight at Vani, who was dumb founded and amazed. "Pia, you are the Pitta type. Right?" Before giving the girl a single chance to refute or agree, Dr Wizard shared a knowing smile with Kavya, who blurted out, "And, I am Kapha type."

"Bang on!" said Dr Ayur wizard approvingly. This made Kavya feel quite pleased with herself.

"All three of you girls have been able to identify your innate personality. And let me tell you that all of you are absolutely right, so congratulations," he said beaming.

The girls let out a collective sigh of relief. Neither of them realised they were holding their breaths and were secretly seeking his approval.

"Now just to confirm what we all have identified, let's discuss your personalities in detail,"

Vani is a typical of Vata type of personality.

"Therefore, her physique (as well as temperament) naturally bears much resemblance to the basic qualities of the air. As air manifests and dominates the being of the Vata type of person, right from birth, the bodily features, as well as mental disposition attributes to the excess of the Vata dosha residing in the body. Subsequently, as is the air (not to forget that this dosha is further made from natural elements of ether and air), so is the individual holding analogous qualities," he explained.

Vata type people naturally reflect the basic traits of the air element.

- Air is ruksha (dry, rough) so the skin and hair are dry and rough just like Vani's. She also keeps getting fissures in the soles of her feet.

- Air is laghu (light) so this individual has a light bone structure. The person would be devoid of fat and mentally, he is a frivolous thinker, with often fluctuating mental states. S/he also sleeps light. Vani has a thin and lean physique. She has dark complexion and her body is devoid of fat.

- Air is shita (cold) so her skin and body temperature remains on lower side and thus she finds it rather difficult to bear cold temperatures seeks comfort in warmth.

- Ether is sukshma (fine, subtle) and this makes the Vata person erratic. S/he jumps to new ideas frequently.

- Air is khara (raw, loose) so the joints, muscles and tendons are devoid of firmness. Sometimes, this person's joints may make a sound on movement.

- Ether is vishada (clear, transparent) and this translates into the Vata person more anxious and easily influenced. All the more, the mental state of Rajas Guna makes the Vata types mentally creative, stimulated and flexible.

"In addition, Vani's nails are rough and get cracked easily and tend to be darker in colour. If you see, her teeth also might be generally uneven, fragile and more prone to dental cavities and plaque. Her voice is rather husky. And if I'm right, and I know I am, Vani is afflicted by occasional depressive moods, emotional fluctuations and indecisiveness," the Wizard finished.

"Yes. I am. But how did you know?" asked a shocked Vani.

"That's the thing with identification. Once we are able to identify a person's type, we are able to learn a great deal about him or her. Here, take these. I've elaborated the characteristics of Vata in detail here. Some of it what we have already discussed, the rest might be additional information," said Dr Wizard.

Sheet 1

Understanding Vata Dosha

Vata governs movement in the body, the activities of the nervous system and the process of elimination. Also, Vata dosha influences the other doshas.

Vata qualities: Cold, light, dry, irregular, rough, moving, quick and changeable. If Vata dosha predominates, movement and change are your dominant characteristics. Vata types tend to always be on the go. They have an energetic and creative mind. As long as Vata dosha is in balance, Vata type individuals are lively and enthusiastic.

Physical characteristics: A person with dominance of Vata would generally be thin—could be tall or short—have a light body frame and rough skin texture. Such people's body parts generally lack stability and show jerking movements. Veins and tendons are more visible. At one time, the person is full of energy and in the other experiences sudden bouts of exhaustion. Hair is often dry and brittle and the voice is hoarse. Vatas typically have dry skin and hair and cold hands and feet. They sleep lightly and their digestion can be erratic.

The Vata type individuals walk fast and generally their joints make a sound on movement. They eat less and prefer food items that are salty or sour in taste. Due to the cold property of Vata, they cannot tolerate cold climates.

Emotional characteristics: Mentally, Vata individuals are a hurried lot. They grasp things fast but soon tend to overlook the subject. During demanding times, they suddenly go into bouts of depression and agony and want to be left alone. Vata types tend to remain on the go with zeal and thrill. They seek new experiences. They get angry quickly but also forgive easily. When Vata dosha is in balance, they happily take initiative and indulge in lively conversations. As a positive trait, those influenced by Vata dosha are significantly creative, action oriented, energetic and flexible.

—End of sheet 1—

Pia is the Pitta Dosha Type or has Pitta Personality

"Now, let's talk about Pia's personality type—Pitta. In people of this disposition, the fire element is predominant. Therefore, the nature of individuals possessing this Prakriti (nature/constitution) show most of the properties of the fire body humour like heat, sharpness, flowing, mobility and being viscous. The salient characteristics:

- Fire is Ushana (hot) so Pitta people are bound be hot tempered. Also, their body temperature remains on the warmer side, making external cool more amiable.

- Fire is sharp and body features generally concur with this quality.

- Fire is flowing, fluid (Drava), which naturally causes more perspiration.

- Fire is mobile (sara). Hence, these individuals remain on the go and often have busy schedules.

- Though you can't hold fire in your hands, it's appears to have a certain oily texture. Fire is Snigdha—oily, viscous—so the skin and hair of people with Pitta have oily texture and radiance.

The mental state of Satwa Guna makes the Pitta type to be more knowledgeable, logical and worldly wise. So, now let's match these qualities with Pia"

"Pia has smooth skin with a yellowish or reddish tinge. Soles of her feet, her palms, lips and tongue have trace of red colour which is slightly deeper than other body parts. Owing to the hot, flowing and oily nature of fire, she is easily afflicted with skin maladies like pimples and acne, freckles and moles. The additional fire in her system makes her generally intolerant to heat and hot climates. There is, by nature, sparse and slow hair growth and her hair shows signs of premature greying. She gives importance to healthy diet intake and is a good eater. Also, personally, she tends to show preference towards cold and chilled foods. As perspiration is profuse and Pia being typical Pitta, finds it rather tricky to bear elevated temperatures and often shows fondness towards use of perfumes, scented talc and deodorants. Due to more heat within, she tends to feel exhausted easily and demonstrates only moderate resistance power. Am I right, Pia?"

The girl was beyond being impressed at the man's ability to surmise correctly. So Pia simply nodded. Once again, Dr Wizard gave them the sheet detailing characteristics of Pitta Dosha.

Sheet 2

Understanding Pitta Dosha

The Pitta dosha controls digestion, metabolism, and energy production. The primary function of Pitta is transformation.

Pitta qualities: Hot, light, intense, penetrating, pungent, sharp, acidic. Those with a predominance of the Pitta principle have a fiery nature that manifests both in body and mind.

Physical characteristics: The body of a Pitta type of person is generally symmetrical with medium body frame and proportionate weight. Pittas are pleasant looking. Their complexion is fair; with the nails, hands, feet, eyes and face showing a tinge of copper. As a Pitta trait, there could be premature greying of hair, early baldness or thinning of hair. Also, the Pittas perspire a lot and have warm body temperature. Sleep is good. When in balance, Pittas have perfect digestion, strong appetite and are energetic.

Emotional characteristics: Pittas have a powerful intellect and a strong ability to concentrate. Ayurveda believes that due to the basic trait of fire, Pittas are mentally sharp, fast, and alert. They are short tempered but calm down just as quickly. Pittas by and large are courageous and heroic. They have a good memory. The Pittas are generally a balanced lot. When the Pitta dosha is in balance, such people are great decision makers and instructors. Generally, Pittas are authoritative, judgmental, sharp-witted, precise, direct and rather outspoken.

—End of sheet 2—

Kavya is the Kapha Dosha type of personality

"Last but not the least; we come to Kavya, the typical Kapha type. Individuals bearing dominance of Kapha dosha display similar characteristics as the properties of the phlegm body humour i.e. coldness, heaviness, viscous, motionless, soft, sliminess and turbidity.

"Thus, all the properties of Kapha (earth + water) come obvious in them.

- Guru (heavy), these individuals are heavy boned with bodily structure that is also on the heavier side.

- Snigdha (oily, viscous), making their skin and hair more oily and supple than others.

- Both earth and water are shita (cool) elements and hence skin of the Kapha types is cool and environmental warmth is much needed.

- Earth has a coarse (Sthula) texture and these people tend to put on weight easily and naturally.

- Earth is also Sthira (stable, motionless), so Kapha types have slow body movements and are more static than other types.

- Water is Slakshma or smooth so the Kaphas have smooth skin and exhibit slow and steady temperament and even poise.

The mental state of Tamas Guna predominates, making these individuals attached to things and also sometimes avaricious. As Kavya has the Kapha dosha or phlegm body humour, which forms her basic individuality, her physical appearance as well as mental temperament would familiarise with the Water and Earth basic elements," said Dr Wizard.

"Typical of Kapha disposition, Kavya has proportionate body and a good stable physique emitting the aura of endurance, strength and stability. At the same time, dominance of phlegm within her system, explains why she tends to put on weight easily. Moreover, her skin is soft, smooth and supple and particularly greasy and glowing. It generally feels cool and gives off bluish radiance. Also, her hair texture is slightly greasy but thick. It can be curly and distinctively dark. She also naturally has a pleasant voice pitch and sound, much like the sound of water. Kavya therefore would be naturally inclined to be a slow and calm person who is never hastened even in her bodily reactions," he said, passing the third sheet detailing characteristics of Kapha Dosha.

Sheet 3

Understanding Kapha Dosha

Kapha qualities: Oily, viscous, cool, Sthula (heavy), Sthira (stable, motionless) and Slakshma.

Physical characteristics: The body is well built, large framed, symmetrical, and attractive. All the body parts are stable and appear to be healthy and full. The Kapha person's complexion is normally fair and rosy, like a lotus, and with the glow of golden colour. Their eyes are large and shiny and show happiness, and the hair growth is dense with black lustre. Kapha types gain weight easily, owing to their sedentary and easy going attitude.

Emotional characteristics: Kapha people are not the hurried type; rather they work with patience and calm. Their voice is strong with a deep tone. They are fertile and lead a healthy life span with less occurrence of disease.

Mentally and emotionally these individuals are of a pious nature, truthful, thankful, and bear a good moral character. They have a good memory, stable nature—they don't change their mind often and are not impulsive.

"As I mentioned earlier, Dosha healing has three portions. Of these, the first one—Self Identification is almost done,"

"We need to classify our physical and mental entity as per the Dosha that shows maximum resemblance in terms of properties, actions, basic physique, timely reactions, likes and dislikes. This indirectly reveals to us the basic constitution and temperament to which we belong.

"We can then take a more serious note of the maladies that the vitiation or aggravation of either of the Doshas is bound to present itself with. Or in many cases, have already caused suffering. It can also be understood that the basic type of Dosha we belong to can be more easily verified as we take notice of the relative ailments. At the same time, they serve as caution to forgo the afflictions that might sooner or later set in and cause unnecessary distress. This means, that tomorrow we will discuss doshas in the light of your health issues. Come prepared," Ayur wizard concluded.

"Now, we're getting somewhere," said Pia as they got out.

"Yes. I'm actually looking forward to this," Vani agreed.

"I told you so. Finally, I'm beginning to get some answers to so many of my unsaid questions. Can't wait for tomorrow to come," said Kavya.

CHAPTER 8

Focus on Health

"Good Morning ladies, without wasting more time, let's get down to discussing your health issues. Reflecting on your health means speaking of both: your physical health quandary as well as your mental health snags," he said looking at the three.

Of the three, Vani was the first to experience the imminence of early aging, though she was impenitently the last person on the earth to acknowledge this (let alone speak it out). But it was increasingly worrying her and she was fed-up of keeping her feelings bottled up. Now, in the class, Vani found an outlet to share her concerns in the hope of finding some remedies.

First, it was her skin. No matter how much she ignored it, her skin was getting drier by the day and showing fine lines. The girl who had now become a middle-aged woman was disturbed and annoyed about it. And it was obvious to all as she kept scratching her arm, leaving a pattern of white lines. The other concern was her receding hairline. She was losing a lot of hair; whatever remained, were brittle and parched tresses.

"Speaking about my hair and skin, I always wanted to confess something to both my friends here," Vani said to Dr Wizard.

"I envy your thick and curly locks," she said turning to Kavya. "I have often thought that if I could confiscate just this one thing from you, I'd feel like a queen," she said.

"And Pia, whenever I have wanted beautiful hair like Kavya, my mind would deliberately hover over your picture. Of all your virtues and good things, I have always yearned for your complexion. I could give away anything for skin like Pia and hair like Kavya," she said.

'Would she barter her slim figure? No way,' mused Kavya to herself.

Not only were early signs of ageing bothering her, but her increasing physical inefficiency too was making her all the more apprehensive.

"In addition, there are some health maladies that are taking their toll. Every now and then, my ankles ache with shooting pain and also my digestion is getting intolerantly gaseous," she divulged. Vani had also been experiencing cramps and sprains every now and then. Of many other things, this was what worried Vani the most.

"I'm not even 40, and I don't know if others are going through this too, but I am experiencing pain in almost my entire body," she said. Both her friends exchanged glances.

Sometimes it was her head, sometimes back, sometimes abdomen or even her teeth. And it made her endlessly brood about what's actually wrong with her? Vani was already an anxious person and worrying about her failing health and fitness made her virtually nutty, restless and irritable.

"I might as well admit to you Dr Ayur wizard, that I seem to be even losing my mental calm. This, at times, leaves me feeling all the more depressed and lonely," she said, breaking into sobs. For the world, Vani pretended to be a fit and robust individual. She even tried to hide the fact that she used spectacles (though everyone knew it). She would hide them in her desk the moment someone entered her cabin. Coffee machine discussions at Vani's office usually revolved around how she was losing her memory as well. Vani hadn't shared her agony and fears even with her husband. But now Harshit had begun to smell the rat. He too was worried about her failing health. But, like rest of the world, he was a silent spectator. Harshit had so many times tried to talk to her but with no outcome.

Pia too was nearing forty and not really happy to acknowledge it. But she was in better health than her friends. "Well, I have for always been somewhat short-tempered but thought would cool down with age. But to my dismay, as I near middle age, I find myself becoming all the more aggressive and impatient," she said. This showed more on her husband as well as on her son. Pia was a strict and disciplined mother who had always made her family's health and fitness her priority. But she was getting increasingly intolerant. Once, when her son joked that his mother is so strict that she would make him wear pullovers even in spring, unlike other 'normal' mothers, she whacked him hard. "This simple sentence enraged me to the level that my face went red, my heart pounded loudly. I just lost my senses and hit my son. But this incident made me to shudder thinking about what I was becoming," she said in a small voice.

It was true. Pia would lose her mental balance even at seemingly small things. Whenever someone tried to mock her, overwhelm her or even deceive her, it enraged her and she lashed out at no matter who it was in front. "One more thing . . . working in the hotel industry was singularly my choice, after nine long years in the same hotel, I am beginning to sense that somehow my colleagues seem to be avoiding my presence," she admitted.

Pia was known to be strict and a tough task master. But sometimes her outrage had interfered with her common sense. A few years back, in a fit of rage Pia had slapped a bell boy in public. The boy was so shamed that he had tried to take his own life. The incident had been the talk of the town for months. Instead of apologising to him, Pia had demanded the boy's resignation. Media intervened and Pia had to openly apologize.

"The incident had left me more furious than ever. I have hated the world for this kind of conduct. I despised being part of the ill-logical, erroneous and immoral humanity. For so many days after the incident, I couldn't calm my nerves. Not at work and not at home. It seemed that even my family had run for the covers and this made me feel forlorn and outwitted," she said and went quiet. There were tears welling up in her eyes. The entire room was enveloped in an uncomfortable silence.

Pia had her reasons for everything she did. She was confident and sure of herself. Yet, the closer she was drawing to her 40th birthday, the more frail and berserk she felt. She was struggling to rationalise the insufferable wrath she felt. She couldn't take it much longer. "Dr Ayur wizard, I also have hypertension, and have always blamed the outside world for it. For the last five years I've been on anti-hypertensive medicines. But now even they don't seem to help. Lately, I've noticed that when things go wrong, my anger is accompanied by something else. My heart starts to hammer loudly and my body heats up as in fever. My digestion has been good, but nowadays I often suffer symptoms of hyperacidity that linger on for days together and my eyes become burning hot," said Pia, perplexed.

Pia also shared about the hot flushes she was experiencing; she feared early menopause. With so many health maladies, her concern about her physical wellness had turned to worry. She often experienced a fall in sugar levels, leaving her hypoglycaemic and weak. It was not the early greying of hair or withering of her skin patches (her doctor had pronounced a disease called Psoriasis and had principally blamed Pia's stressful and edgy nature for it) that was a nightmare for her, but her real apprehension was her son. "My husband is such a lenient father and I fear it would spoil our child," she said, digressing from the topic. What began as a discussion about her health issues was now becoming a chat about an anxious mother. Dr Ayur Wizard understood that underneath her confident composure, Pia had begun to crack—her health afflictions were scaring her.

Kavya, the third friend, also in her late thirties, confessed that for the past one or two years, she has been increasingly feeling good for nothing. Both her friends agreed that, they too have been noticing the drastic change in Kavya. She had become an altogether different person now. The bubbly, plump girl, who was full of life and vigour, had now become obese and inert. For days on end Kavya would sit brooding over her fate trying to understand what was going wrong with her. The more she thought, the more she ate and the more she ate, the more she thought. This had become a vicious cycle with no exit in view. It was as if she was trying to fill some void inside her. But her face showed as if she wanted to say something but was hesitating.

"Kavya', Dr Ayur Wizard said coming over to her.

"You can discuss anything you want in class. No one will judge you or say anything to you," he said in a voice full of compassion, gently placing a hand on her shoulder.

Kavya could just not contain herself anymore. The excruciating pain she felt in her heart was unbearable, she had been walking around with that knife in her chest for too long. "I am childless," she said in a low voice. There, she had said it.

Vani's hand flew to her mouth. Pia just blinked in shock and said, "what!" Kavya had not breathed a word about this to anyone, not even her best friends. The disbelief on her friends' faces turned to sympathy for their friend. Vani got up and hugged her friend. And Kavya started whimpering like an injured pup as tears flew unabashed down her chubby cheeks. She was inconsolable.

Finally, Dr Ayur Wizard asked her friends to leave Kavya alone. This was actually needed as she had suffered the agony silently all these years and had spoken about it openly for the first time. This gesture actually helped and within a few minutes, Kavya was taking long breaths all by herself, gathering courage to come out with her story.

"Well, I want to confess this in front of you all today that I have not been blessed with my 'own' child. My daughters, who mean the world to me, were actually born to my husband's sister. She had a difficult delivery and could not be saved. She left these beautiful twin girls behind. It was then that Rahul decided that we take care of the little infants who were left without a mother. Since then, we have publically pronounced ourselves as their parents. I really love my girls," said Kavya turning to Dr Ayur Wizard, "I am so attached to them and they make me feel complete," she said. "But deep inside I know that I'm childless," she said a fresh stream of tears flowing down.

Before adopting the girls, Kavya and her husband had left no stone unturned for remedies and treatment for a childless woman. Being a prominent doctor, Rahul had used all his considerable resources, getting her the medical attention of the best doctors in India and abroad. Alas, none could figure out what was wrong with Kavya. All her laboratory tests and sonography reports were normal. But it was suggested to her that she shed some weight. "I have tried my best to lose weight. But it seems to be the most difficult job on earth," she said looking at Dr Wizard, who smiled at the unspoken question in her eyes.

Kavya told them that in the early years of her married life, weight loss seemed like a petty issue and she paid little heed to it. But now in her late thirties, it was increasingly becoming a huge problem. Kavya was seemingly a peaceful and quiet person but internally it was as if she nurtured a dormant volcano.

Being overweight was a sure debacle for Kavya, but there were more heath afflictions that seemed to bother her. She often experienced bouts of allergic cough and nasal congestion, which would aggravate with the slightest triggers such as change in the season. During those episodes, she struggled with breathlessness. "Doctors always put me on nasal puffs and anti-asthmatic drugs, which only seem to add to my weight. I'm really fed up of these medicines. Dr Wizard. My husband is a doctor, but I refuse to believe his professional opinion that these medicines and nebulizers are the only way out for me. There surely has to be something else that can cure me without making me feel being dull, disoriented and drowsy. Why the hell does he refuse to understand my plight!" It was an outburst no one present knew how to control. "This has led to many fights between us", she continued. "Though I have to admit that Rahul is the best thing that happened to me," she added hurriedly.

"And linked to this is another of my gnawing concerns. My declining health and also my embarrassing external appearance have made me possessive about my husband. Every time he leaves town for a seminar or conference, I am consumed by the fear that he might find someone better than me. And I end up eating all the more," she admitted.

A pin-drop silence followed. After a beat, Dr Wizard cleared his throat and smiled at Kavya. "Thank you Kavya for opening up your heart in front of us. And with Kavya's story, now we all know what ails each one of you, not just physically but mentally as well. Though all three of you are suffering from loss of health, your ailments are distinctly different from each other. While Vani has erratic digestion and psychological problems,

CHAPTER 9

What Causes Disease?

Dr Ayur Wizard explained that imbalance causes disease.

"In Ayurveda texts, the same is explained in Sanskrit as: 'Rogastu dosha vaishamyam doshasam yamarogata' (AH Su 1/20)"

He explained that according to Ayurveda, an individual can only enjoy the fruit of health in case all the three Doshas viz. Vata, Pitta and Kapha remain in their natural balanced state (in properties and functions). When either of the Doshas becomes vitiated, it results in formation of disease or disorder in the body or mind.

"What causes imbalance of Doshas," asked Vani?

In answer to her question he explained that there are three basic reasons for any discrepancy in the basic Doshas of the body to occur:

- Decrease in the functions as well as properties of one or more Dosha.

- Increase in the functions as well as properties of one or more Dosha.

- Opposing functions and properties of one or more Dosha.

It has been stated in Ayurveda text that the Dosha gets vitiated or aggravated when an individual with a particular prakriti or constitution—vata, pitta or kapha—tends to follow aahara and vihara (diet and lifestyle) similar to his basic Dosha type. This may be justified by the simple principle of 'like increases like' Or "Sarvadasarvabhavanam samanayam vridhikaranama" as mentioned in ancient Ayurvedic texts.

Aggravation of a Dosha is bound to throw it out of kilter. This later on takes the form of a malady.

Dr Wizard explained that as a dominant sign, Vata causes pain; Pitta results in a burning sensation and Kapha leads to swelling. Ayurveda believes that a disease that has emerged due to vitiation of a single dosha is considered to be easy to cure. Whereas the ailments arising out of imbalance of more than one Doshas are intricate to cure and the disease or disorder in which there are signs of vitiation of all the three Doshas is said be rather incurable.

He then went onto explain imbalance of Vata Dosha in detail.

As per Ayurveda, Vata imbalance accounts for 80 types of diseases and disorders. Therefore an individual showing characteristics of Vata Dosha is prone to these following maladies.

- Muscular and nerve pain.

- Pungent taste in the mouth.

- Recurrent indigestion or slow digestion.

- Constipated or hard stools.

- Hoarseness of voice.

- Cramps and convulsions.

- Excessive thirst.

- Easy fatigue and progressive weakness.

- Shaking and shivering sensation.

- Roughness and tearing in the skin and fissure formation.

- Occasional feeling of deafness.

- Diminished immunity.

- Sleeplessness and recurrent headaches.

- In severe cases, paralysis and Paresis.

Like I mentioned earlier, "Vata easily falls out of balance with anything that is undertaken (diet and lifestyle) that resembles the basic characteristics of the Vata dosha or the air humor in the body," he explained.

So tell me, what are the characteristics of Vata?" he asked Vani.

"Vata is Ruksha—dry, rough," she offered.

"Correct. Hence, intake of arid and dry foods and living in dry weather conditions, will lead to Vata imbalance," he explained.

Similarly, Vata is Laghu or light. Hence, eating meagre meals, fasting or holding on to hunger or eating foods that supposedly have high air content such as aerated drinks too will aggravate Vata in one's body.

Since Vata is Shita or cold / cooling, intake of cold and frozen foods and living in cold environment is not recommended.

He then listed the other Vata characteristics and their corresponding lifestyle habits that aggravate Vata.

- Sukshma or fine, subtle, penetrating. Restraining on the natural urges and often changing moods with less of mental concentration on a single subject.

- Khara or raw, loose. Rushing with body parts, uncontrolled speech, excess physical exercise forceful on the joints and bones.

- Vishada or clear, not viscous, transparent. Sudden intense changes in life, seasonal changes, mood swings.

- The mental discrepancy of Rajas Guna to remain in state of anxiety, nervousness and apprehension also vitiates Vata.

- Vata gets naturally aggravated during old age, in the late evenings, during cloudy skies, after taking meals and in the rainy season.

- Intake of food items that are dominant in bitter, pungent and astringent tastes.

- Habitual suppression of natural urges like urge to pass stools, to urinate, to pass wind, belching etc.

- Exposure to cold climates.

- Ignoring, delaying or forgoing sleep.

- Keeping mentally alert or anxious due to un-accountable fears.

- Taking up routines of long brisk walks or heavy exercises.

- Working without rest and ignoring the body's need to take a break both physically and mentally.

- Talking a lot and giving very little or no rest to vocal cords.

- Accidental traumas like falling from a height or fractures.

"Now, the next logical question would be what are signs of Vata imbalance?," Dr Wizard continued. "This sheet lists them all," he said passing around sheets of paper.

Signs of Vata imbalance

- Rough skin with occasional dry itching; cracked nails and brittle hair.

- Constipated motion and more flatulence.

- Digestion and appetite patterns become varying.

- Tremors, muscle twitching, numbness.

- Disturbed sleep, mood swings, fears.

- Body and joint pains are moving and piercing and feel better on pressing.

- Aversion from cold, and a desire for hot foods and environment.

- Continuous feeling of lethargy or lassitude.

- Restlessness or impatience.

- Frequent muscular cramps and body ache.

- Mentally, there are obvious signs of frequent inability to memorize. Fearfulness, nervousness and sometimes depression might prevail.

"When the Vata dosha becomes imbalanced, the physical maladies that would generally manifest in the body are weight loss, constipation, hypertension, arthritis, weakness, restlessness, indigestion and sleep afflictions. Also, when imbalanced, mental reactions would be that the Vata individual becomes rather prone to worry and anxiousness and often suffers from insomnia and disturbed sleep. The Vata person would easily become disillusioned and feel inundated and stressed. In any such situation, he often remains perplexed with thoughts like 'What is wrong with me?', he explained further. Imbalanced Vata may result into failure of retention.

Vata or the air body humour when aggravated has a tendency to be yet more perilous than the other doshas. This is because of the erratic and unstable natural trait of this dosha. Vata types need to be more cautious as this particular dosha type could be effortlessly thrown out of balance.

"As I mentioned, Vata imbalance results in 80 ailments. These are:

1. Nakha bheda or cracking of nails

2. Vipadika or cracking of soles of the feet

3. Padashula or pain of the feet

4. Padabhramsha or steps not falling at the right place while walking, flat foot

5. Padasupta or numbness of feet.

6. Vatakhuddata or pain in the hip joint.

7. Gulphagraha or sprain or stiffness of the ankle

8. Pindikovestana or cramps in calves.

9. Gridhrasi or sciatica

10. Janubheda or bow legs

11. Januvilesha or Knock knees

12. Urustamba or stiffness or paralysis of the thigh

13. Urusada or pain in the thighs due to atrophy of thigh muscles

14. Pangulya or lameness or deformed foot

15. Gudabhramsa or prolapsed anus

16. Gudarti or pain and tenesmus in the anal region

17. Vrishnotksepa or pain in the testis or in the scrotal area.

18. Sophasthamba or stiffness of the penis.

19. Vanksanabha or tension in the groin.

20. Sronibheda or pain around the pelvic girdle

21. Vibheda or loose motions

22. Udavrata or paralysis of the intestines

23. Khanjatva or lameness

24. Kubjatva or hunch back

25. Vamanatva or dwarfness

26. Trikagraha or arthritis of the sacro-iliac joint, neuralgic pain in the sacral region

27. Pristhagraha or stiffness of the back

28. Prasva vamarda or pain in the chest along with difficulty in breathing

29. Udaravesta or gripping pain in the abdomen

30. Hrinmoha or heart block, heart failure or cardiac inactivity

31. Hriddrava or palpitations, tachycardia

32. Vakshaudgarsa—Rubbing pain in the chest

33. Vakshauparodha or damage of the thoracic movement

34. Vakshastoda or stabbing pain in the chest

35. Vahushosha or atrophy of the arm

36. Grivastambha or stiffness of the neck

37. Kathoddhvamsa or hoarseness of voice

38. Hanubheda or dislocation of the jaw with severe pain

39. Manyastambha or spasmodic contraction of neck muscles causing stiffness of the neck on one side.

40. Osthabheda or pain and tearing of the lips

41. Akshibheda or Pain in the eyes

42. Dantabheda or tooth pain

43. Dantashaithalya or looseness of the teeth

44. Mukhatva or dumbness

45. Vaksanga or impaired speech

46. Kshayasyata or astringent taste in the mouth

47. Mukhshosha or dryness of the mouth

48. Arasagyata or loss of taste

49. Grananasha or Anosmia

50. Karnashoola or pain in the ears

51. Ashabdashravana or Tinnitus

52. Ucchaisruti or hard of hearing

53. Bhadirya or deafness

54. Vartma samkocha or retraction of the eyelids

55. Vartma stambha or Rigidity of eyelids

56. Akshiyudasa or eyeballs raised upwards eyelids

57. Timira or partial loss of vision

58. Bhruvyudasa or eyebrows raised upwards.

59. Shankabheda or headache with pain in the temporal area, migraine

60. Lalatabheda or headache with pain in the frontal area.

61. Siroruk or headache

62. Kesabhumi sphutana or fissures on the scalp, dandruff

63. Ardita or facial paralysis

64. Ekanga Roga or Monoplegia

65. Pakshavyadha or Hemiplagia

66. Sarvanga Roga or paralysis, paraplegia

67. Akshepa or clonic convulsions

68. Dandaka or tonic convulsions

69. Shrama or excessive tiredness

70. Vepathu or tremors

71. Jrimbha or yawning

72. hikka or hiccups

73. Bhrama or giddiness

74. Vishada or state of unhappiness

75. Atipralapa or delirium

76. Rukshata or dryness

77. Parushya or hardness, Harshness

78. Syavaruna dhasata or Dusky red appearance of body or part of the body

79. Aswapna or loss of sleep

80. Anavishthita chitva or mental instability

He then outlined imbalance of Pitta Dosha.

Pitta Dosha is believed to cause 40 types of diseases and those of the Pitta type might in their lifetime often come across ailments like:

- Infection and inflammation of various organs.

- Profuse perspiration with foul smell and dark colour and putrid smell of urine and faces.

- Feeling of restlessness, irritation, anxiety and intolerance for hot things.

- Inability of the liver to perform well causing occasional acidity, gastric ulcers and anorexia.

- Recurrent headaches with a burning sensation redness of the eyes.

- Occasional convulsions and hysteria.

- Burning sensation and redness anywhere in the body as in the eyes.

- Weakness of the sense organs particularly vision afflictions like impairment of vision.

Anything that has similarities with the fire dosha aggravates it and causes imbalance.

- Since Pitta is ushana or hot, having foods with hot potency and staying in warm environment for a long time aggravates this dosha.

- Since Pitta is Tikshana or sharp, severe emotions and also following an intense, spicy and potent diet aggravates it.

- Since Pitta is Drava or flowing, remaining emotionally intense and always on the run is not advised.

- Since Pitta is Sara or mobile, keeping superfluous busy schedules with little physical and mental respite aggravates it.

- Since Pitta is snigdha or oily and viscous, intake of oily and fried foods aggravates it.

- The mental state of Satwa Guna is predominant in Pitta, which makes the fire person highly intellectual. Yet, imbalance draws in when the mental positive virtues are overpowered by Pitta emotions of criticism, over judgment and antagonism.

- Naturally, the Pitta Dosha gets aggravated in the middle age, in the middle period of the day i.e. afternoons and middle part of night, while taking meals and in autumn season.

Other things that aggravate Pitta Dosha include:

- Eating foods that are predominantly sour and bitter.

- Hot foods and beverages, high salt diets and intake of chilies, fried foods.

- Alcoholic or fermented drinks.

- Over-indulgence in sex.

- Excessive anger and episodes of jealousy and high expectations, and also fretting over nominal issues.

Signs of Pitta Increase

- Yellowish skin, eyes, urine and stools.

- Disruptive sleep or insomnia.

- Gastric symptoms of acidity, loose bowels, nausea, vomiting, metallic taste in mouth.

- Skin boils, acne, urticaria, bleeding gums.

- Hunger pangs and low sugar levels. Increased liking for cold foods and sugar craving.

- Emotionally aggressive, anger, jealously & irritability.

- Burning sensation anywhere in the body.

- Vertigo and superfluous tiredness.

- Acidic eructation and bitter taste in the mouth.

- Natural craving for cool things.

"The mental attributes of failure of demarcation between right or wrong which may take form of uncertainty. Episodes of unconditional disapproval and irritation prevail. The Pitta imbalanced person may show signs of becoming jealous, critical and over condemnatory. Mainly the mental imbalance in Pitta types would be the failure of discrimination," he added.

Explaining it further Dr Wizard said, "When Pitta falls out of balance, the fiery component becomes obvious. Pitta imbalance often shows with the individual being short-tempered and confrontational. When out of balance, Pitta reasons for physical implications like skin rashes, burning sensations, peptic ulcers, excessive body heat, heartburn, and hyperacidity. When a Pitta type individual is imbalanced, his response would be "What did you do wrong?"

"Lifestyle measures like excessive anger and episodes of jealousy and high expectations, and fretting over nominal issues, over-indulgence in sex, taking foods with hot potency and staying in fairly warm environment for a long time tend to aggravate the Pitta dosha. Also, keeping superfluous busy schedules with no or very little physical and mental respite," he said.

Imbalance of Pitta is responsible for forty ailments:

1. Osa or heat stroke

2. Plosa or scorching of the skin

3. Daha or burning of the skin

4. Dawathu or burning sensation in sense organs like eyes etc

5. Dhumaka or feeling of fumes coming out from the head

6. Analaka or acid eructation

7. Vidaha or burning sensation in palms, soles of the feet

8. Antardaha or burning sensation in the entire body

9. Amsadaha or burning sensation in a part of the body

10. Ushmadhikaya or very high body temperature

11. Atisweda or excessive perspiration

12. Angasweda or sweating in a part of the body.

13. Angagandha or body odour

14. Anga vardhna or fissures on the surface of the body

15. Shonitakleda or pernicious anaemia

16. Mamsakleda or degeneration and softening of the muscular tissues

17. Twagdaha or burning sensation in the skin

18. Mamsadaha or burning sensation in the muscles

19. Twagavadarana or cracking or scaling of the skin

20. Charmavadarana or deep cracking of the skin

21. Raktakotha or putrefaction of the blood

22. Rakta Pitta or bleeding from body pores

23. Haritatwa or greenish colour of the skin

24. Nilika or blue moles

25. Kaksha or herpes

26. Kamala or jaundice

27. Raktamandala or red wheels on the skin

28. Haridratva or yellowish colour

29. Tiktasyata or bitter taste in mouth

30. Putimukhata or mouth odour

31. Trishnadhikya or excessive thirst

32. Atripti or insatiable hunger

33. Ashyapak or mouth ulcers

34. Galapaka or throat inflammation

35. Akshipaka or conjunctivitis

36. Gudapaka or proctitis of the anal region

37. Medhrapaka or inflammation of the penis

38. Jivadana or haemorrhage

39. Tamahpravesa or unconsciousness, fainting

40. Haritharida netra, mootra varchastva or greenish and yellowish colouration of the eyes, urine and faeces.

Explaining imbalance of Kapha Dosha Dr Ayur Wizard told them:

"Kapha Dosha accounts for 20 types of diseases and a Kapha type of a person may suffer from the following maladies," he said, listing them on the whiteboard.

- Diseases of the respiratory tract like repeated colds and cough.

- Excessive production of phlegm, saliva, urine and feces.

- Occasional constipated stools and impaired digestion.

- Feeling of drowsiness and lethargy.

- Sweet taste in the mouth or variations in tastes.

- Itching and whiteness of skin.

- Feeling of nausea and vomiting.

- Poor metabolic rate and tendency of developing disorders like obesity and diabetes.

- Tendency to sleep more than average.

- Feeling of coldness and rigidity coupled with heaviness and stiffness in joints.

As in earlier cases, following a diet and lifestyle that resembles the Kapha Dosha characteristics aggravates it.

Kapha is heavy (guru), So intake of heavy diet or overeating.

Kapha is oily and viscous (snigdha). So, eating fried, oily and unctuous foods aggravates it.

Kapha is turbid, gelatinous (pichhila). So intake of slimy, viscous foods and beverages aggravate it.

Kapha is cold, cooling (shita), therefore cold environment and cold foods and drinks like ice creams aggravate it.

Kapha is coarse (Sthula). Hence the tendency of a Kapha person to hold on to fixations and emotions leads to problems.

Kapha is stable / motionless (Sthira). So leading a sedentary life, sitting or resting for too long, especially sleeping during day time leads to problems.

Kapha is smooth (Slakshma). So, using smooth textures, living easy, carefree attitude in daily routine causes its imbalance.

The mental state of Tamas Guna predominates in this particular Dosha. When this takes form of negative mental emotions like possessiveness and acquisitiveness, Kapha plunges out of balance.

"The Kapha Dosha is believed to show natural aggravation in the younger age, during early mornings, during the start of a meal, during snowfall and in the spring season," explained Dr Wizard. Other things that cause imbalance of Kapha include:

- Foods those are more cold, heavy and unctuous.

- Excess intake of food that are sweets; milk and milk products.

- Little or no exertion of the brain powers.

- Less or no exercise routine.

- Less physical and vocal activity and leading a lethargic and sedentary lifestyle.

SIGNS OF KAPHA INCREASE

- Pale skin, nails, eyes, urine and stools.

- Excessive sleep, lethargy, heaviness.

- Water retention, swelling, weight gain.

- Heaviness after food, excessive saliva, loss of appetite with sweet taste in mouth and occasional sensation of nausea.

- Cold, cough with phlegm, sinus congestion, breathlessness.

- Dull, lack of enthusiasm and desires

- Mental imbalance of Kapha—failure of determination.

- Easy weight gain.

- Increased oiliness of skin and hair.

- Excessive phlegm formation, especially during the early mornings.

- Increased susceptibility to sinuses and respiratory system disorders.

- Morning congestion.

"On psychological matters, emotions of possessiveness and over-attachment are apparent. Incapability of willpower sets in making the Kapha person all the more dormant and inert. Sometimes Kapha imbalance might promote greed and acquisitiveness," he explained. Mental imbalance in Kapha type is the fear of determination.

I want you to remember the following about Kapha imbalance, even though I may have said this earlier," he said and went on to state the following:

- Foods that are more cold, heavy and unctuous, and increased intake of sweets or foodstuffs that are sweet in taste, milk and milk products would cause easy aggravation of Kapha dosha. Ayurveda states that of the six basic tastes known to human tongue, the phlegm humor tends to exacerbate by more intake of sweet, salty and sour tastes.

- In everyday lifestyle, activities like sleeping during the daytime, keeping a relaxed and carefree attitude as well as less exertion of the brain powers, less or no exercise routine. Similarly, leading sedentary life, sitting or resting for too long causes Kapha imbalance and also to be holding on to fixations and emotions does more harm by eventually throwing Kapha out of kilter.

- The mental state of Tamas Guna predominates in this particular personality. When this takes form of negative mental emotions like possessiveness and acquisitiveness, Kapha plunges out of balance. The Kapha imbalance may mentally result into self-questioning as—'Why have I been wronged?' Failure of determination may result due to Kapha dosha imbalance.

The 20 ailments resulting from Kapha Imbalance are:

1. Tripti or feeling of full abdomen

2. Tandra or drowsiness

3. Nidradhikya or excessive sleep

4. Staimitya or feeling of wet cloth covering the body

5. Gurugatrata or heaviness of the body

6. Alasya or feeling of lethargy

7. Mukhamadhuraya or sweet taste in the mouth

8. Mukhasrava or excessive salivation from the mouth

9. Shleshmodgirana or mucous expectoration

10. Malashyadhikya or excessive formation of faecal wastes

11. Kathopalepa or excessive mucous production in the throat

12. Balashaka or tiredness, loss of strength

13. Hridayoplepa or feeling of wet cloth tied to heart region

14. Dhamanipratichaya or thickening or dilation of the blood vessels

15. Galaganda or Goitre, tumour in the neck

16. Atisthaulya or obesity

17. Sitagnita or suppression of digestion

18. Udarda or urticaria

19. Shwetava bhasata or Paleness of the skin

20. Shwetamutra netra varchastva or whitish colour of the eyes, urine and faeces

"Remember, that an ailment transpires from imbalance. And imbalance results mainly from improper diet and inappropriate lifestyle. And the reason of all this is also apparent as alike qualities attract and also augment. When Dosha aggravation causes imbalance within the body system, then signs of imbalance set in which later on in the process take form of a disease," he said, concluding the session for the day.

CHAPTER 10

Step Two: Self-Understanding

The previous day the girls were pretty kicked to learn about the cause of disease and dosha imbalance. And were looking forward to learning more the next day as they were beginning to understand how the Doshas were affecting their lives. For instance, Pia now understood why having too much oily food troubles her. So the next day, the girls were early in class and were busy discussing with each other the various signs and symptoms that they were experiencing, when Dr Ayur Wizard walked in.

With a huge smile he said, "You'll be glad to know that we have successfully completed the first step of self-identification."

"Yay!" shouted the three in accord.

"And," he continued after the noise died down, "we are well into the second step. Does anyone remember what the second step is?" he asked, looking at the three.

"Self-understanding," said Vani almost jumping out of her seat, which made the others laugh.

"Bang on! Step two is Self-Understanding. As is evident from the name, this step will test how well you understand your own self."

This perplexed the girls once again. Of course, each one knew herself quite well, what was there to test? More importantly, what was there to understand more? They exchanged puzzled glances and started whispering among themselves. The hum of conversation grew louder as Dr Wizard turned his back to them to retrieve something from his briefcase. They hardly noticed that he had returned and was standing in front of them, keenly observing them, waiting patiently for their conversation to get over. When it was clear to him that it wasn't going to happen anytime soon, he cleared his throat and called them to attention.

That got their alertness and all fell silent again. He then passed them a set of yellow coloured sheets and said, "Now girls, this is not home-work for you, but you have to complete this right here and right now in front of my eyes."

That surprised the girls, who couldn't decide what was worse, homework or an in-class assignment.

Ignoring the looks on their faces he continued, "This is important because this small exercise will help you overcome your next hurdle and you will be able to understand yourselves better, in the right way. This is all you will be doing in the class today. Take your time but I want the mission accomplished before all three of you leave the premises." Dr Wizard sensed discomfort among his class and realised that one of the three girls will soon throw a tough question at him. He therefore decided to take the lead. "I want no more discussions on the topic or complaining behind my back. Once, again, I don't mind if you take half an hour, two hours or the whole afternoon for this. It's up to you. But by the evening leave your answer sheets on the table and only then can you go home," his tone discouraged any retorts. The message was clear enough for the three girls and they hurriedly began to fumble with the yellow sheet of paper now lying just in front of each of them.

This sheet was different from the Self—Identification questionnaire they had filled up recently. This one was the Self-Understanding Sheet along with 'Do-it-yourself' project, which appeared to them more or less like a Self-Assessment mission that they were yet to accomplish. This yellow colour sheet contained subparts along with blanks which they had to fill.

As soon as Dr Wizard left the class, Pia was the first one to break the silence. "My God, another lengthy paper for us to answer! This time, it is class work. This is too much.

I wonder how much more exams we have to undergo in this class. If all three of us agree, we can raise a voice against this kind of conduct. After all, we are not school kids, are we?" When there was no answer, that's when Pia realised that she had been talking to herself. Both her friends were already engrossed in their paper work. For a moment, this surprised her and almost enraged her, but then she realised that there must be something in this paper that was keeping both her friends so occupied. And she for one, didn't want to be a laggard. So reluctantly, she turned her attention to the task at hand.

It was almost an hour before the three finished their 'Self-assessment sheets'. So when Dr Wizard appeared, from wherever he had gone, none of them had noticed. They were totally oblivious to his presence. He grabbed the opportunity to catch a shut eye. As expected, Kavya took the longest, which gave Dr Wizard a chance to extend his snooze sitting head-down on his table.

He was awakened by the sudden volume of the girls chatting among themselves. He woke up to find that all three had finished their papers and were now busy comparing notes.

"Ok, ladies. I see that you've completed the sheets. Kavya, would you please collect them for me and bring them here," he said.

Here's what the sheets contained.

Do it Yourself—Self Understanding Project

Vani's Self Understanding Sheet

My personality

(Present a picture of yourself that depicts your characteristics)

My assets: I am slim, tall and do not gain weight easily.

My limitations: I have dry skin generally and tend to have rough, brittle hair. I have a dark skin tone and my voice has heavy pitch.

My character

(Behavioural Aspect and Forbearance)

My assets: I am quick and versatile. I can take rapid decisions. I am active and my mind keeps throwing up new ideas, innovations and fantasies.

My limitations: I remain hurried and am always on the go. Being talkative comes to me naturally. Many a times I don't seem to be able to hold myself back or slow myself down.

My attitude

(My response and basic nature)

My assets: I am mostly full of ideas, vibrant and energetic. I love to dream and actually avoid taking life seriously. I get motivated easily and try to stay clear of any argument and binding. Also, I love change and don't like sticking to one thing for long.

My limitations: I can be impulsive and unpredictable at times. I can easily get stressed, which further makes me feel like the world has come to an end for me. Trivial things can make me anxious and exhausted.

My wellness

(My health and maladies)

My assets: I would say my health is OK. I generally feel fine and enthusiastic.

My limitations: I have sensitive and dry skin, nervous headaches and digestive disorders keep bothering me every now and then. Also, I feel weak and drained-out often. And I keep getting episodes of joint pains or muscular cramps. I am intolerant to cold, windy weather and generally have cold hands and feet, particularly during winters.

My diet chart and eating habits

My assets: I'm not really a foodie, but I keep munching on small portions of food throughout the day. As for eating habits, I can finish my meal quickly while others around me seem to be taking double the time.

My limitations: My digestion gets affected easily. Whenever I vary from my normal eating—if I eat more or less than usual—I suffer from indigestion and bloating. I have noticed that certain foods like ice creams, cold drinks, fried foods, chillies and spicy food do not suit me, though I'm so quite fond of them.

My lifestyle

(Everyday living and routine)

My assets: I can remain really active and on the go. I am basically a lively and versatile person.

My limitations: Often, I tend to become overactive or over talkative and then feel loss of energy. I have also seen that if I brood on some issue or problem for long, I suffer from anxiety and I lose my sleep.

Pia's Self Understanding Sheet

My personality

(Present a picture of yourself that depicts your characteristics)

My assets: I have a proportionate body with symmetrical build and height. My skin is fair, supple and has a natural glow.

My limitations: My skin is oily and so I am prone to pimples, acne and moles. Considering my age, my hair seems to be greying early and have become sparse. Also, I am easily susceptible to sun burns.

My character

(Behavioural aspect and forbearance)

My assets: I'd like to think I'm smart, amicable and inventive. I tend to be a passionate and dynamic person. Some would call me a go-getter. Also, I can be easily relied upon. I have leadership qualities and have good communication skills.

My limitations: I can be judgmental and easily irritable. I tend to lose my temper easily and can even be aggressive. I have noticed that I can be rather fiery (as my reaction to a stimulus), intense, judgmental and also competitive.

My character

(Behavioural aspect and forbearance)

My assets: I am intellectual and witty, can solve problems on the go and have a great aesthetic sense.

My limitations: I can be irksome and extremely linear in my thinking, especially when I am troubled or tensed up.

My attitude

(My response and basic nature)

My assets: I am logical, reliable and honest. I find cooler climates and environments relieving.

My limitations: I flare up easily because I'm a perfectionist and I just cannot stand unruly people and situations.

My wellness

(My health and maladies)

My assets: Generally, the state of my health is optimal. Also, I am blessed with a good digestion and metabolism.

My limitations: I have noted often that I am prone to falling ill during late spring and summer. It feels like my body heats up as I have high temperature. During such episodes I have excessive thirst and also perspire more. The sweat is often foul smelling. I have also noticed that many times, I have a bitter taste in my mouth for no apparent reason.

My diet chart and eating habits

My assets: My hunger pattern is good—rather too good at times. I feel I have wonderful digestion and generally am comfortable eating most of foods if taken in moderate quantities. Most amicable diet for me is juicy, succulent fresh fruits and fruit juices.

My limitations: Spicy food and even fried food just doesn't suit me—they trigger acidity. I can feel real hunger pangs and tend to feel drained if I have to go hungry for long.

My lifestyle

(Everyday living and routine)

My assets: I can remain reasonably active, and generally find it easy to follow a timetable or a lifestyle routine.

My limitations: I sleep light and get disturbed easily. Hot climatic conditions don't suit me and I get irritated and angry soon.

Kavya's Self Understanding Sheet

My personality

(Present a picture of yourself that depicts your characteristics)

My assets: I have a clear and fair complexion and have thick black hair that has certain bounce.

My limitations: I am large framed and thus have a rather hefty look. I tend to gain weight easily.

My character

(Behavioural aspect and forbearance)

My assets: I have good stamina and general resistance. I'm generally admirable and loving. I stick to my words, do not change my mind easily, I am trustworthy and loyal.

My limitations: Sometimes I feel lethargic. I also feel greedy. I am naturally a possessive person. My actions and reactions are slow, even my digestion takes more time as compared to others.

My attitude

(My response and basic nature)

My assets: I am a soft-spoken person and take time to react. I am slow and steady in my reactions and responses.

My limitations: I can be extra slow and inert at times. Fixation to ideas and situations come to me naturally. I take more time than most people to analyse and take to a situation. But once I do, I stick to it.

My wellness

(My health and maladies)

My assets: I am generally healthy, other than the problem of phlegm.

My limitations: I tend to be vulnerable to sickness during spring and late winters. My illnesses tend to revolve around congestion, fluid retention or excess mucus. My ailments can be short listed as obesity, drowsiness, laziness and loss of memory. I suffer from recurrent episodes of nasal congestion, coughs and colds with excess phlegm formation. In addition, I can't be very active; in fact I feel drowsy and lethargic at most times. This makes me prone to being over-weight. Also, I often have a blocked nose and suffer sinusitis related headache.

My diet chart and eating habits

My assets: I can eat almost all kinds of foods very easily and with proper hunger. As for my eating habit, I eat slowly and my digestion is fine although it takes more time.

My limitations: Whenever I over-eat, my digestion gets affected almost every time. At such times there remains lingering sweetness in my mouth and my abdomen feels full. This happens frequently and makes me uncomfortable. I have a sweet-tooth which also causes me to gain weight easily.

My lifestyle

(Everyday living and routine)

My assets: I am generally a relaxed person. My sleep is good and I go through my day with patience.

My limitations: I can be very slow and lethargic. Getting up early during mornings is an impossible task for me. Sticking to same schedules day-after-day sometimes makes life feel monotonous.

CHAPTER 11

Moving Towards Clarity

The next day which was pre-decided by the Wizard for sorting out all sorts of queries and probes regarding the subject of Dosha Healing, was here now. The three girls were in the class much before he entered and Dr Wizard took his own sweet time getting to the class or so it seemed to the three friends who were dying to ask him questions and get their doubts cleared. "Hello, there. I'm sure you're ready with your questions. So who wants to go first?" he asked.

All three raised their hands, Vani and Pia even pushed each other doing so like little girls, while Kavya, always the balanced one, did so with a quiet smile. "Kavya, shoot," he said.

"How does Ayurveda define wellness or illness?" asked Kavya.

"Although by now you all know about this very well, yet for the purpose of revision, I'll answer this one again. Ayurveda categorises all individuals as per the basic dosha that is dominant in them. Vata, Pitta and Kapha are the three basic doshas or body humors that are actually the root cause of both wellness and illness. Mind it ladies, I repeat, doshas are responsible for both your sickness as well as your health. As per the science of Ayurveda, a person is healthy only as long as the doshas are in equilibrium, and an imbalance in the same leads to disease. As has been specified by Charka, the originator of Ayurveda,

Rogastudoshvayshamyam doshsamyamarogta.

"This means that whenever there is imbalance in dosha (body humor), it causes disease; while the balanced dosha bestows the bounty of health.

"You may be naturally a Vata type or Pitta type or Kapha type or even a combination type. Actually combination types are more common, but at the same time, when you go through the body-mind questionnaire in detail, you can still come out with a dominant dosha in there, which all three of you have successfully determined," he said grinning at them.

'And can't a person have all three doshas?' It was Pia who put across the query.

"Yes of course young lady, but these kind of individuals are rather sparse in existence,"

"What is the need for Dosha Healing?" Pia asked.

"If we want to lead a good life, it becomes rather mandatory to determine the basic dosha (Vata, Pitta or Kapha) that reigns within us as it determines both our constitution as well as our temperament. It is indeed a delight to be able to understand and accept oneself at such a basic level. And it also helps us understand those who touch our lives. Like for instance all three of you childhood friends are so much different from each other. As you know Dosha healing actually segregates people according to the basic elements of Ether, Air, Fire, Water and Earth, each of which has its distinctive natural properties and characteristics. Vani is Vata type having more of air and ether within her. Pia on the other hand is mainly fire dominant and makes the Pitta type of personality. Whereas Kavya has more of water and earth elements and thus has the Kapha type of prakriti. Do you see the divergence now? Vani is generally unsettled, Pia is intense and Kavya is relaxed, and all this is Natural manifestation. Learning this and understanding this, helps us live a healthier and aware life,"

"Is Dosha Healing really a science?" asked Vani.

"Yes it is, but not in the sense that it is done in a laboratory. Something doesn't have to be modern to be a science. Dosha Healing is the oldest healing science originating from Ayurveda, which itself is 5000 years old," he said a bit annoyed.

"How can Dosha Healing help me?" asked Kavya.

"Once you are able to ascertain your innate dosha, you can understand yourself better and eventually take care of yourself in accordance with the dominant dosha that makes up your basic personality. The harmonising dosha bestows on you natural health and wisdom. At the same time, it is a great aid for you to enjoy lifelong wellbeing, joyful spirit and attractive body," he said.

"Does that mean Dosha Healing can help me become beautiful?" asked an astonished Vani.

"As I just said Dosha Healing helps you immensely to discover and enhance your natural beauty, wisdom and wellbeing. This is because once you are able to identify and concur with the basic dosha that supports your system, you can more easily decide about the right diet and lifestyle for yourself. And as you balance and harmonize your dosha, then acquiring as well as maintaining internal and also the external beauty is easy. Besides there are dosha-specific beauty aids to help you. For instance, using potent oils is great for Vata types, whereas Sandalwood pastes or Rose water therapies work best for Pitta types, and honey based preparations suit the Kapha types," the Wizard replied.

"Can Dosha Healing make a person healthy? Pia asked.

"Health is nothing but non-existence of disease. It's like a see-saw . . . when your health goes down, the disease goes up, and vice versa. Therefore, all you need is to focus on maintaining the balance, and this is where Dosha healing basically comes into play. Dosha healing aids both as preventive as well as curative therapy. Especially if you are aware about the dosha imbalance that could more easily impinge your system. I'm sure you all remember that Vata types are more prone to be influenced by 80 types of ailments, Pitta types may be affected by the 40 kinds and Kapha types need to consciously surpass the 20 types of Kapha diseases. Does that answer your question?" he asked looking at Pia, who nodded in response.

"Dr Wizard, now I'm clear about how Dosha healing can help me with my health, but I want to know if it can help me improve my relationships and compatibility?" This came from Vani.

"A good question, but a tricky one," he said.

After a few minutes of contemplating the question, he said, "Visualise Dosha Healing as your aid in all spheres of life. To be compatible in your relationships and associations, be it at home, at work or at social engagements, calls for awareness both about your own self as well of the individual with whom you are connecting. All the three dosha types (Vata, Pitta and Kapha) are influenced by different mental states. And once you get the hang of Dosha healing, you will come to recognise the basic Dosha personalities of those close to you. You will know their basic mind-set, and realise that their behaviour is merely a natural manifestation of the dosha. You can then consciously attempt to either ignore or accept the inert nature and attitude that is the play of dosha dominance. That's how Dosha Healing aids to amend liaison first with your own self, and then with all others with whom you are connected," he answered.

Clearly impressed by his answer, the three nodded in agreement.

"Can Dosha Healing help me lose weight?" asked Kavya

"Dosha Healing helps regain balance. When you are in physically balanced state, your body weight also has to be proportional and symmetric. Anything extra that is sticking to your body, and that is not required by your body, is toxic matter. Therefore, obesity is rightly one of the most dreaded and distressing lifestyle diseases today. But to answer your question, yes obesity can be tackled with dosha understanding and self-awareness. Kapha type of people have a natural tendency of weight gain and hence need to be more firm with themselves both in terms of consciously and strictly following the recommended diet as well as lifestyle. If they do so, then certainly they can have a proportionate and fit body.

"Can Dosha Healing help me in developing my business or dealing with job complications?" asked Pia.

"Are you thinking of leaving your job in hospitality and starting something new Pia?" Vani teased.

"I have been thinking about it. But that's not why I asked. I really want to know," she replied seriously.

"Dosha healing is part of Ayurveda, the science of life. Therefore, it deals with all aspects of one's life—be it office, business, health or relationships. Once your mind-body is in balance, it's easy to think all the more rationally. Business dilemmas, dealing with colleagues, leadership demands all can be taken care of when you learn to think outside-the-box. Ayurveda philosophy of Dosha Healing can help corporations significantly enhance their productivity and creativity by aligning employees' roles and responsibilities with their individual physical and mental energy patterns or the dominant doshas within the individuals. In fact, I do work with several corporates doing just this enactment for their staff," he said.

"How can Dosha Healing help me become more productive?" asked Vani.

"The objective of Ayurveda is to keep the three Doshas properly balanced not just for the benefit of your body, but also your mind. Indeed, if your Vata is in balance, you can be creative and super-active but if Vata is in excess, you will experience anxiety and frustration more often. Similarly, if your Pitta is balanced, you act as a focused, intelligent, and passionate person but if imbalanced, Pitta will fill your mind with anger and make you judgmental. Also, if your Kapha is in balance, you may be much grounded and act as great decision-maker and manager but if imbalanced, Kapha can make you sluggish and inflexible and too possessive and also attached to your ideas and plans. To be more productive, all you need is to keep your doshas balanced," explained Dr Wizard.

Before anyone could ask, Kavya cut in, "You said earlier that Dosha Healing helps in interactions with colleagues . . . does it also help when devising a business strategy?"

"Yes, it does. When you are designing a business strategy, you need to understand that your team's collective dosha or the energy pattern will be shaped by the doshas of its individual members. Ideally, all you need to do is to form a team with balanced dosha personalities. This means when you are making a group and assigning different work, see that you get together the right mix of people with Vata (creative and energetic), Pitta (passionate and determined), and Kapha (grounded and cautious) dosha types,"

"Wow," said Pia, impressed.

"Can Dosha Healing help me in day-to-day things like de-stressing and/or getting a good night's sleep?"

"Of course, it can. In fact, Ayurveda Dosha Healing has specific recommendations for this. For example, if you are Vata type, sleeping on your left side aids in right nostril breathing, which is warm and thereby balances the cold Vata. For Pitta types, sleeping in moonlight or amidst cool air and showers, or in cool dark shade will do you good. Also, if you have more Phlegm or Kapha in your system, sleeping during daytime is a strict no-no. Once you are able to manage the right sleep requirements for yourself, sleep will soon be a non-issue," he explained.

He noticed that Kavya had become silent. She was lost in thought. Snapping his fingers in front of her eyes Dr Wizard said, "Kavya, is there anything that you want to ask? You seem to be brooding over something,"

"Oh! Sorry. No there's nothing," she said quickly.

"I think there's something you want to ask but you are hesitating. It's ok, we're all friends here, you can ask what you like," he said.

"Does Dosha Healing also help in matters of intimacy . . . . I mean in a person's sex drive? Does this ancient healing science also relate to some distressing conditions like infertility and impotency?" she asked in a low tone.

"The ancient healing science of Ayurveda is really vastly accommodating in all the spheres of life. Sex is a very personal subject and each of the dosha types would have different considerations and endurance regarding it. Therefore, a thorough understanding of the innate dosha that determines your basic existence also plays important role in defining your sexual needs and gratification; and also the medical problems arising due to the same," he said.

"In case of Vata types, you must remember that owing to the Vata dosha dominance in your system, your sexual needs and also capacity of enjoyment is somehow meagre. Vata types are generally creative, unpredictable and wary. They naturally have a low interest in sex and more often they indulge in the act mainly for communicating their love to their partner. Therefore, satisfying relationship and performance, while indulging in the act, would help Vata types relieve their anxiety and provide them with much needed warmth to balance their innate dosha. The right timings and time-tables are important for Vatas, and thus planning the routine ahead of time both physically as well as mentally, would do them good," he said.

He then informed them that with regards to physical ailments relating to the reproductive system, Vata is most likely to have sex related problems like impotency and sterility or lack in conceiving due to anxiety, dryness, low body weight and disturbed Apana vayu (the type of Vata residing in the lower portion of the body).

"Dosha healing would help you understand that in case you are Vata type, you need to save your desire as well as energy. Slowing down and resting as and when needed, would help you enjoy the act. Also, mentally you need to keep away from unnecessary apprehensions," he explained.

Addressing Pitta types, he said that people in this category generally find moderate sexual desire and limited approval among the opposite sex. As and when the Pitta imbalance sets in, the positive qualities of Pitta types (ambitious, passionate and warm) may be surpassed by the competitive and judgmental nature of Pitta dosha.

"This is where you need to be cautious, as this may hamper your sex life and leave you rather unsatisfied and jaded," said Dr Wizard.

He explained that as per Dosha Healing, if you are Pitta type, you need not vent your emotional energy out more often by indulging in the act of physical respite. Also, as more involvement in sex results in Pitta imbalance, you need to keep yourself in moderation and refrain from being too vigorous and heated up during the act. Pitta types may suffer from impotence or infertility due to excessive heat forming up within the reproductive tissues. Restricting being in the act more often, especially during summers and in warmer climatic conditions is needed for Pitta types.

As for Kapha types, the scenario would be altogether different. These individuals have good amount of trapped-in energy in their systems. Therefore, sex life for them would be moderate-to-good. In accordance with the innate Kapha Dosha, the emotion as well as desire for love making would generally be on the rise. Kapha is enduring, balanced, determined and fostering. Also, Kapha persons are naturally very sensual and are regarded to be basically sturdy and fertile individuals, and would generally not be facing sex and reproduction issues like impotence and infertility.

"But if you understand it well, Dosha healing could make you aware that the same Kapha that keeps you stable and passionate could also make you very attached and avaricious at times. In this case, you could be unnecessarily spoiling your sex liaison with your partner. Being aware and not yielding to such emotions is necessary for you. Moreover, Ayurveda counsels the act of sex also as a form of exercise, especially for the Kapha type personalities. Therefore, your sex drive as well as frequency is well justified," Dr Wizard explained.

He then asked the girls if there were more questions. But perhaps speaking about such a personal issue had left their mind blank so no one said anything. There was silence in the class.

"Ok so. I take it that you ladies are done with your questions," he said and got nods in reply. "I hope that you now have more clarity on the concept of Dosha Healing. Just in case, if you do have more questions or doubts, feel free to mail me even after the workshop is over. I'll revert within two working days," with that he concluded the day's session.

CHAPTER 12

East V/s West

Although the three had resolved most of their queries, they still had this feeling that they were missing on something. That there were still things they didn't have answers to. They were clearer on the subject and had collectively put forward as much questions that came to their minds, yet there was something more they were in the lookout. Perhaps, they were seeking validation that that Ayurveda and Dosha Healing that seemed to have solutions to all their problems, does indeed work.

As if reading their mind, Dr Wizard said, "I know that the ancient wisdom of Ayurveda sounds too good to be true. And that's why there is a lot of scepticism surrounding it, which isn't wrong. Yes, the ancient wisdom hasn't been developed through 'modern-day research and development', but those who developed it did their own research. It's an experience that has journeyed ages," he clarified.

"Has anyone heard about Personality factors by Raymond Cattell?" he queried.

When he got blank looks he told them that Raymond Cattell was a British and American psychologist. He was known for his work on Cattell's 16 Personality Factors. These are well researched and accepted.

"I am now going to show similarities between Cattell's 16 Personality Factors and the three precise magnitude of Dosha Healing (Vata, Pitta and Kapha personalities) which allays the discord between the western and eastern approaches to mental health conceptualisation," he said.

"Let us consider three distinct factors of neuroticism, conscientiousness and emotional stability," he said.

He explained that these traits may also be observed in the unique psycho-physiological constitution (dosha diagnosis or prakriti). Vata types would score high in neuroticism than Pitta and Kapha types, whereas the Pitta types would score higher in conscientiousness than the Vata types or Kapha types. And yet, the Kapha types would score more in emotional stability than the Vata or Pitta types.

According to the modern-day science, we are believed to relate to particular traits or dispositions. These personality traits had been earlier described by psychologist Gordon Allport in more than 4,000 words. After this, Raymond Cattell analysed the detailed list of varied personality traits, and used a statistical technique known as factor analysis to identify traits that are related to one another. By doing this, he was able to reduce his list to 16 key personality factors. Cattell had developed an assessment based on these 16 personality factors. The test is known as the 16 PF Personality Questionnaire and is frequently used today in the western world, especially for employee testing and selection, career and marital counselling.

"You know that the personality types laid down by Ayurveda refer not just to body types but also emotional make-up. And that all three doshas are present in each one of us. Cattell too believed there is a range of personality traits and each person contains all of these 16 traits to a certain degree, but they might be high in some traits and low in others.

"Without going into the mystifying details and arguing between the ancient and modern concepts of Personality traits, let me try to make it evident that the tool of dosha identification and understanding which provides you with the analogous and comprehensive relevance, also essentially helps you to fit in the Personality factors (as expressed in modern science).

"Here, I'm citing for you the personality trait list which describes 16 personality dimensions defined by

Cattell. Please see for yourself and understand how the well-known personality factors of the western world, are similar to our basic dosha traits of Vata, Pitta and Kapha,"

1. Abstractedness: Imaginative versus practical. Vata type will score maximum.

2. Apprehension: Worried versus confident. Maximum for Vata types.

3. Dominance: Forceful versus submissive. Pitta type would score maximum.

4. Emotional stability: Calm versus high strung. Highest for Kapha type.

5. Liveliness: Spontaneous versus restrained. High for Vata type, good for Pitta type.

6. Openness to change: Flexible versus attached to the familiar. Maximum for Vata types, least for Kapha types.

7. Perfectionism: Controlled versus undisciplined. Pitta scores highest.

8. Privateness: Discreet versus open. Kapha types show maximum trait, least for Vata.

9. Reasoning: Abstract versus concrete. Pitta shows max trait, Kapha is low here.

10. Rule consciousness: Conforming versus non-conforming. Pitta has max, Vata has least trait.

11. Self-Reliance: Self-sufficient versus dependent. High for Pitta types.

12. Sensitivity: Tender-hearted versus tough-minded. High for Vata types, good for Kapha types

13. Social Boldness: Uninhibited versus shy. High for Pitta, Low for Kapha types

14. Tension: Impatient versus relaxed. High for Vata, low for Kapha types.

15. Vigilance: Suspicious versus trusting. High for Vata, low for Kapha types.

16. Warmth: Outgoing versus reserved. High for Pitta, low for Kapha

He then explained that this relative association can prove an important bridge between eastern ancient healing science of Ayurveda and the modern medicine concepts of the western world. The 4000 personality traits by Gordon Allport or the 16 personality factors by Raymond Cattell may be well summarised within the three Dosha types of Vata, Pitta and Kapha.

The harmony between the two is evident. The test of 16 personality factors composed of choice questions and the personality traits are represented by a range and the individual's score falls somewhere on the continuum between highest and lowest extremes. Same would be the case of your assigned doshas. According to Ayurveda Dosha Healing concept, Vata dosha is reported to be responsible for a quick response or rapid movement, Pitta dosha is described as the dosha which is responsible for metabolic activities, whereas Kapha dosha would be generally static and inert, and thus shows in the various Personality factorization.

Dr Wizard's purpose behind bringing the relevance of the Personality factors was that the girls could understand for themselves that although the western personality constructs might not align absolutely with the Ayurveda Doshas, they lend substantial support to the likelihood of correspondence between the eastern and western models of healthcare, basically taking in consideration the perspective of mental health.

Dr Ayur Wizard finally found the feeling of confidence in the faces of his students. Are you convinced about the credibility of Ayurveda now?" he asked.

The girls were totally convinced about the authenticity of Dosha healing. All three were silently musing on how 4000 or 16 traits of human personality as portrayed by modern science today could fit in only the three doshas that were acknowledged more than 5000 years ago. Leaving them pondering, Dr Wizard announced that the class was adjourned.

CHAPTER 13

Step Three: Self Care

When the girls came in the class the next day, there was a mixed feeling in the air. For, it was their last class. And though initially they were reluctant to join, they had now come to like their interactions with Dr Wizard, benefitting from his wisdom and learning about Dosha healing, and more importantly, about their own selves. Knowing about *doshas* and personality types had helped them make sense of so many things that earlier baffled them. They had come in early and the mood was sombre. So when Dr Wizard had turned up, he was surprised to see them sitting quietly, notebooks open and pens at the ready.

As usual, he greeted them with a warm smile and began, "So my dear young ladies, we have come to the concluding session of your familiarity with Dosha healing, the ancient wisdom science of healing through Ayurveda. By now, all three of you have not just identified but also understood your basic personality or the '*Prakriti*'. You now have the answers to the basic questions about yourself . . . questions like 'What/Who am I' and 'Why am I so?' among others."

The three friends continued to listen in rapt attention and made no attempt to interrupt Dr Wizard, who was amazed that he had spoken without a single query, commotion or disruption by his audience. He deliberately took a long pause, watching his solemn students.

"We've covered steps one and two i.e Self Identification and Self Understanding. I'm sure you are clear on both the aspects by now. Any questions? Is everything clear to you?" This time, there were nods but not one spoken word.

"Ok, then. We have reached the last leg of our journey, last step—Self Care. This is the final chapter of your book on Dosha Healing," he said, looking at the three.

There was a note of accomplishment in Dr Wizard's voice, as if he had scaled Mount Everest and was all ready to pitch his triumph ensign. "Oh yes, here we are now at the concluding part of the entire counselling session that we worked together on," he said reiterating what the girls already knew.

"I want to give my heartfelt thanks to all of you as you have been a wonderful audience, tolerant and enduring," he said, clearly taking the three by surprise. This, they hadn't expected.

Vani was all-smiles already; it was a moment of personal achievement for the girl. Since she was the first to respond, Dr Wizard first turned to her. "Vani, I want to declare, you were fairly modest and patient during the entire class, and I owe special obligation to you," he said nodding in appreciation. Vani mumbled a thank you.

"My dear Pia," he said turning to the girl, who almost blushed and forget to frown at being addressed as 'my dear'. "I want to say that your sense of positive apprehension and inquisitiveness helped me delve deeper into the subject." Pia remained impassive, all the while wondering whether Dr Wizard's tone and words conveyed genuine appreciation. Or was he pulling her leg?

But Dr Ayur Wizard had turned his attention to Kavya, "Of course, the sweet and nubile Kavya, whose innate forbearance and zeal has helped us remain persistent. She helped bring in compassion into the dreary sessions," Kavya almost bowed in response.

"Now, I once again ask for your complete attention. We all know that after this session on Dosha Healing, you will return to your respective lives and worlds. But this time, you have a potent tool with yourself that will always be there with you. Now, you would be able to discover, appreciate as well as accept both the positives as well as negatives not only in yourselves, but also in other people (or circumstances) you deal with. Dosha Healing is going to be your great support for nurturing this quality. I say this with certainty that comes out of experience," said Dr Wizard, looking straight into each one's eyes.

"Just a few moments back, I had said that we have come to the final chapter of 'Your book' on Dosha Healing. Did you hear me ladies? I said 'Your' Book. This journey is like a book and you are the author, editor as well as publisher of your individual book. I have given you something and I anticipate you to return the favour," he said. Perplexed, the three exchanged glances, wondering what he expected them to do.

"It's simple," he said, "All you need to do now is write down your own story. You are now your own guide as well as healer. Please don't forget young ladies that you and only you know yourselves too well, all your worries, queries and now even solutions. Better than any other person living on this earth. Does anybody differ from this opinion?"

None of the three friends had the courage to counter his statement, not even Pia, for a change!

"Then it's settled. All three will sit separately and prepare the basic approval and recommendation sheet for yourself, taking into consideration your virtues and vices, dos and don'ts, why's and why not's. Now, now don't worry young ladies, this is surely the last time that you are being made to go through this exercise, and I'm sure you can do this as well as you've done the other! You will, right?"

Dr Wizard waited for a whole minute for them to say something. The silence was shattered with a nervous laughter from Kavya. It was weird, and the other two found themselves helplessly imitating and giggling, without rhyme or reason. Dr Wizard continued, "This is not a joke. I'm serious. And here comes another twist in the story, my dears. Now wipe off the drops of sweat on your foreheads and look into the papers on your desk with your eyes wide open. All you need to understand is this:

According to Ayurveda science of Dosha Healing, it is important to eat your diet as well as indulge in daily activities that have a balancing effect upon the dominant Dosha within your being and also that will pacify (stabilise) the Dosha that has become excessive or aggravated.

Before they could realise, three crimson sheets of paper were swiftly placed before each one of them.

Chapter 14

Suggestions for Self

The girls now focussed completely on the sheets in front of them. They knew by now that Dr Ayur Wizard would permit them to leave no stones unturned in giving their best. The Self-care task sheet was clearly divided into two portions of diet and lifestyle, and to their surprise had already been completed by Dr Wizard!

There were squeals of laughter as relief as well as gratitude flooded through them. They were saved from the tedious work of filling in the details. But one glance at Dr Wizard's serious face told them that the Self—care sheets before them now called for sombre contemplation. Also they noticed that at the end of each assignment, there were a few four lines left blank and mentioned along with these lines were words written in bold alphabets—SELF CARE FOR ME

Self Care Project

Vani's Self-Care Diet Recommendation Crux Sheet

As you are Vata type, you must remember that your basic dosha has the properties of being drying, cooling and light. Therefore, the diet that would suit you and balance Vata dosha needs to be oily, warming, and fairly heavy. The best tastes to pacify Vata are sweet, salty and sour. Also, you need to take less of the foods that are pungent, bitter, or astringent.

Going on fasts more often, skipping meals or irregular timings for food aggravates digestion discrepancies of Vata types.

To balance the lightness of Vata, eat moderately heavier quantities, but refrain from overeating.

All sweeteners pacify Vata and may be taken in moderation. The basic properties of your food need to be warm, nourishing and unctuous.

You may feast on a variety of fruits, which are somewhat heavy and sweet like dates, apples, bananas, papaya, grapes, sugarcane, avocados, mangoes, apricots, plums, berries, coconut, figs, grapefruit, orange, lemon, melons, peaches and pineapples.

As for your vegetable intake, you are advised to eat less of ground tubers. Have more greens, broccoli, asparagus, beets, fenugreek, bitter gourd and carrots. You need to eat less raw vegetables and fruits; they are better had lightly steamed or cooked, roasted in low oil or sautéed in ghee.

Dried fruits, sprouts, peas and cabbage tend to produce gas and hence their intake should be kept at a minimum.

In cereals, red rice, wheat, black gram and raggi are good.

As for drinks, you may have fresh buttermilk with invigorating and digestive spice powders like black pepper and asafoetida (which are Vata balancing). Also, warm and mildly spiced soup is good for you.

Kitchen herbs, spices and condiments are recommended for you. It's good if you include asafoetida, large cardamom, fennel, carom seeds (*ajawain*) and black pepper in your daily diet.

Have pulses or dals only in moderation; reduce intake of Bengal gram.

You particularly need to avoid dry and cold foods as well as carbonated drinks.

Fats and oils are fine for you as these help reduce Vata. Warming oils like sesame seed oil or mustard oil or even olive oil are good. So, include them in your diet.

Dairy products pacify Vata. Therefore, milk and milk products like curd, paneer (cottage cheese), butter, buttermilk and ghee are recommended in your everyday diet. Milk is easier to digest for you when warmed or heated before drinking.

If you are non-vegetarian, you can have fresh, organic chicken, fish and other seafood, and eggs.

DIET SELF CARE FOR ME

(Vani decides)

Diet recommendation: I need to take food in moderate quantity, but with more frequency. Grazing on small portions of diet is beneficial for me. I need to feast more on foods like milk, green vegetables, eggs, fish, almonds and moderately fried foods. I understand that as my digestion is delicate, warm foods that are only reasonably heavy would suit me. And my diet should consist of foods with sweet, salty and sour tastes.

Restriction: I need to avoid being very choosy about food. Keeping my belly empty or overstuffed will adversely affect my digestion. Eating quickly and talking while eating is something I need to learn not to do. Chilled drinks, too much of chillies and spices, as well as raw food is not good for me. Have to remember moderation is the key for me.

Vani's Self Care Lifestyle Recommendation Crux Sheet

Remember that the basic properties of Vata are cold, light, irregular, dry, and always changing. Therefore, to balance Vata, you need to make choices that bring warmth, stability, and consistency into your life. As you are Vata dominant personality, stress and erratic everyday living leads to your Vata force becoming imbalanced. The erratic and moving nature of Vata or the air also keeps your mind racing, which further leads to anxiety and insomnia. As and when Vata imbalance sets in, following a set time-table is the best recourse for you. You need to deliberately slow down, take time to meditate, not skip meals, and get to bed earlier at night. A regular lifestyle routine helps to ground the erratic Vata.

For the Vata types, sleep pattern needs to be organised and followed. Try to go to bed before 10 pm and rise in the morning by 6 am.

Also, you need to follow an exercise and yoga routine every day. Remember, you may experience periods of high energy, but you also tire easily. Light exercises that enhance balance and flexibility are best for you. You may try walking in fresh air, light cycling and light aerobics. Pranayama and deep breathing techniques of Bhastrika, Kapalbhati and alternate deep breathing would be of help. Take care not to push yourself too much and exceed the limits of your energy. This again causes Vata imbalance.

As for seasonal intervention, care is needed during rainy season, which naturally vitiates vata. Also, you need to pay more heed when the weather is cold and dry as in winters. Wear adequate clothing and preferably keep your head covered. During the cool weather, sip ginger tea many times in a day.

Everyday massage is good for you. Use warm and heavier oils like sesame seed oil and mustard oil.

Also as for your sex life, both desire and energy needs to be saved. Again, moderation is the key.

Be certain that your bowels move regularly on a daily basis.

Avoid getting emotionally upset by small triggers. Try to keep involved and better take up a gentle hobby to remain distracted of unnecessary apprehensions.

Aroma therapy is another help. Inculcate sweet, heavy and warm aromas using lavender, saffron and cinnamon oils.

Use warm colors in your clothing and environment such as earth colors, pastels, browns, and warm yellows.

Important message for you is follow routine and remain balanced as much is doable and comforting for you.

LIFESTYLE SELF CARE FOR ME

(**Vani decides**)

Recommendation: More of relaxing and regular routines need to be practiced. Meditation and Yoga asanas, especially the Pranayama or deep breathing techniques and Massage therapy would be of assistance. I should make a time table for myself.

Avoidance: Keeping on the go, being very talkative, over-anxiety, late nights and over exercising need to be passed up or discouraged religiously.

Pia's Self Care Diet Recommendation Crux Sheet

As you are basically Pitta type with more of fire in your system, aggravation in Pitta dosha heats the body as well as mind and therefore cool foods and liquids and maintaining mental cool will help you. Foods with sweet, bitter, and astringent tastes are recommended and yet the other three tastes—salty, sour and pungent need to be restricted in your daily diet.

Remember not to skip meals and do not wait until you are starving before you eat.

Milk and dairy are good for balancing the heat of Pitta. Ghee or clarified butter is greatly recommended in Pitta diet.

Although Vegetarian diet is good, you can occasionally have chicken, turkey and fresh water fish. Sweet is one of the suggested tastes for you. Therefore, all sweeteners may be taken in moderation. Deserts prepared from sugarcane juice and powdered jaggery are advised.

Cooling, soothing and moderately heavy oils like coconut, olive and sunflower oil are recommended as they help pacify Pitta. Warm oils like sesame seed oil and mustard oil may be avoided.

Sour, fermented products such as yogurt, sour cream and cheese should be used sparingly as sour tastes aggravate Pitta.

Increasing the intake of sweetened fruit juices, cold drinks, *sherbats* and coconut water helps.

Also in fruits, reduce intake of sour fruits like citrus lemon, orange and berries and also unripe fruits. Sweeter fruits such as grapes, melons, coconuts, avocados, mangoes, pomegranates and plums are recommended.

You need to reduce the intake of chillies, spices and condiments. Pitta types need only to use seasonings that are soothing and cooling. This would include coriander, cardamom, cinnamon, and fennel. Hotter spices such as ginger, asafoetida, black pepper, fenugreek, clove, salt, and mustard seed should be used sparingly. You may masticate some fennel seeds after meals so as to cool the acids in the stomach.

As for vegetables, most gourds, cucumber, spinach, pumpkins, broccoli, sweet potatoes, potatoes and green leafy vegetables are good. Eat less tomatoes, garlic, hot peppers, eggplant, garlic and radish. Restrict intake of horse-gram and flat beans.

Your choice for grains in diet may include red rice, wheat, barley, sooji and oats. Eat less corn, rye and millet.

You need to sustain normal blood sugar levels and for this eat at regular intervals and avoid skipping meals.

DIET SELF CARE FOR ME

(Pia decides)

Recommendation: Milk, butter, apples, avocado, watermelon, melon, rice and whole grains, ghee (clarified butter) are good for me as also colder foods and drinks. It's better I don't fast often.

Avoidance: I need to stay away from or at least cut down on my intake of spicy food and alcohol, caffeine, salty and oily foods.

Pia's Self Care Lifestyle Recommendation Crux Sheet

As for the basic traits, Pitta types have the personality analogous to the natural properties of Pitta dosha viz. hot, sharp, sour, pungent, and penetrating. Therefore, to balance the Pitta, you need to incorporate things and activities that are cooling, sweet, and stabilizing in your daily life.

Pitta relaxation and sleep is a must and therefore you need to take more care as your sleep can be affected easily. Avoid keeping lights on at bedtime, sleep more relaxed and preferably on your right side. This encourages left nostril breathing, which is cooling and soothing for you.

Similarly some pranayama techniques like Sheetali and Sheetkari Pranayamas are recommended as they are cooling. Deep breathing is also suggested through left nostril. Your exercise pattern or walk pace should not be too vigorous.

You need to spend time amid nature and keep your mind relaxed and rejuvenated as much is possible for you. Take walks in the woods and along natural bodies of water. Keep plants and fresh flowers in your home and office. Leisure walks in the moonlight and during early mornings in the fresh air is especially suitable for you.

Be careful in autumn season. This is because autumn vitiates pitta and therefore needs more concern.

As you have more of fire in your system, you have to make effort in keeping your mind cool. For this, you may spend time with friends who are not competition for you.

Compassionate massage with soothing and cooling oils like coconut or olive oil and crèmes is good for you.

Pitta types may indulge in aromas that are cooling and sweet like sandalwood, rose, jasmine, mint, lavender and fennel during an aroma massage. Or use the same as aromatic candles in your vicinity.

Favour cooler colours in your clothing and environment such as blues, greens, and silver. Blue, violet and indigo are meant for you.

Engaging in laughter therapy would be of help as it is stress relieving. Practice laughing many times each day as you have to de-stress occasionally.

Follow a regular daily routine allowing some free time for self every day. Be careful not to create unnecessary time pressures for yourself.

LIFESTYLE SELF CARE FOR ME

(Pia decides)

Recommendation: I must try and maintain mental cool, relax and chill more often.

Avoidance: Warm climate conditions, much sun and saunas are not good for me.

Kavya's Self Care Diet Recommendation Crux Sheet

Kapha dosha is heavy, oily and cold, therefore to balance it, the diet of Kapha type people needs be light, dry, hot and potent. Foods with pungent, bitter, and astringent tastes are recommended for pacifying Kapha. You also need to cut down on the foods with sweet, sour, and salty tastes.

Your digestion is slow and heavy and therefore it is advised that you have your largest meal at lunchtime. A gap of three hours between dinner and bedtime is a must.

Your fruit intake needs to be less to moderate and should preferably be during daytime. Lighter fruits like apples, pears, pomegranates, cranberries, and apricots are meant for you. Reduce heavier and highly sweet fruits like dates, coconut, bananas, figs, avocados, pineapples, oranges and peaches.

In vegetables, most gourds, onion, ginger, garlic and radish are fine for youbut reduce consumption of sweet and juicy vegetables such as sweet potatoes, tomatoes and potatoes.

All spices except salt are pacifying for Kapha. You are free to use pungent spices like pepper, cayenne, mustard seed, and ginger in your diet.

It's good if you include hot and spiced soups in your everyday diet. Drinking hot ginger tea also helps stimulate slow digestion and sharpen the overcast taste buds. Take your tea with less milk in it and with less or no sugar.

Fasting is recommended for Kapha types. Your fasts need to be strict with more liquids that include fresh vegetable and fruit juices, lemon water and bland vegetable soups. Fasting once a week would do you good.

Milk and milk products need to be minimal in your diet, though you may have a little ghee, low-fat milk and low-fat yogurt.

You can have more wheat, barley, millet and corn in cereals and less oats, rice and black gram.

Although indulging in sweet tastes is a strict no-no for you as this aggravates your dosha, you can have honey as it best pacifies Kapha.

You need to consciously cut down on fats and oils in your diet. Use only small amounts of extra virgin olive oil, ghee, almond oil, corn oil, sunflower oil, mustard oil, or safflower oil.

The kitchen herbs good for you are **Holy basil, curry leaves and mint.**

Reduce intake of dried fruits and nuts.

As for non-vegetarians, organic white meat chicken, turkey, eggs, and seafood are okay. You should reduce your intake of red meat.

You must avoid cold, creamy foods, deserts, carbonated and frozen foods.

Kapha types need to remember to maintain proper gaps of at least three hours between the meal times because of slow digestion, and also the diet needs to be potent and full of energy to invigorate the sluggish gastric fire.

DIET SELF CARE FOR ME

(Kavya decides)

Recommendation: Apples, apricots, peaches, plenty of fresh vegetables, chillies, onion, chicken and fish are good for me.

Avoidance: Sweet foods, fatty foods, dairy products and heavy starchy foods. I also need to maintain a gap of three hours between meals.

Kavya's Self Care Lifestyle Recommendation Crux Sheet

Since Kapha is inherently cold, heavy, and static, keeping yourself stimulated by the means of active lifestyle is recommended.

Follow a daily routine, ideally awakening by 5am each morning. Keep yourself more active and energetic during the Kapha time of 6 to 10 am. Sleeping during the day is strictly forbidden

You can indulge in all Pranayamas and Yoga poses energetically. Kapha types are prone to congestion and will benefit immensely from using Ayurvedic Neti pot that helps nasal cleansing. Deep breathing is advised mainly through the right nostril because of its warming effect.

Kapha types are comfortable in warmer environments. You need to keep yourself warm and avoid cold and dampness. Avoid exposing your nose, throat, and head region to cold winter air.

Be more talkative with friends where you can relieve and vent your emotions as well as held up energy.

Stimulating, deep tissue or dry massage will help stimulate circulation.

You may also indulge in dry massages and performing self-massage.

Exercise has to be an important part of the daily routine of Kapha types. This is the best way to avoid stagnation and accumulation of toxins in the body. You may go for long and brisk walks, running, bicycling, swimming, aerobics, and engage in competitive sports. The idea is to utilise the stored energy and sweat out to release toxins.

Stimulating and warm aromas are good for you like basil, eucalyptus, cloves, camphor, cinnamon and marjoram.

Your choice of colours also needs to be warm and bright. The colours that would suit you more are yellow, orange, and red.

Of all the seasons, spring vitiates Kapha the most. Also, keep yourself warm in the colder season and climatic conditions.

Another lifestyle help for Kapha types is to remove clutter often not only from your body in terms of detoxification and mind by meditation, but also in your space and surroundings. You need to preclude accumulation as much is possible even if this means clearing the muddle from your home, office, car and other physical spaces.

LIFESTYLE SELF CARE FOR ME

(Kavya decides)

Recommendation: Active lifestyle, keeping on the go both, physically as well as mentally is important for me.

Avoidance: Insufficient exercise, over-eating, excessive dependence on a loving relationship isn't good for me. Also, I need to keep clutter away from every sphere of my life.

Sheet 1

Favourable Diet Chart

Diet	Vata Type	Pitta Type	Kapha type
Favorable Tastes	Sweet, salty & sour	Sweet, bitter & astringent	Pungent, Bitter & astringent
Properties	Warm, nourishing, unctuous	Cold, potent, heavy	Hot, potent and light diet
Action	Hot	Cold	Hot

Fruits	Apples, bananas, papaya, grapes	Less citrus lemon, orange etc	Less to moderate, only in daytime
Vegetables	Less of ground tubers, take less raw vegetables	Most gourds, cucumber, spinach, green leafy vegetables	Most gourds, onion, ginger, garlic, radish. Less potatoes
Cereals	Red rice, wheat, black gram, raggi	Red rice, wheat, barley, *sooji*, oats	Wheat, oats, less of rice, black gram
Drinks	Buttermilk, warm soup	Fruit juices, cold drinks, coconut water	Hot & spiced soup, water boiled with ginger, pepper, lemon. Add honey

Milk products	Curd, *paneer*, butter, buttermilk, ghee	Ghee is good	Only in moderation
Spices & condiments	Moderate intake	Less	More is needed
Kitchen herbs	Asafoetida, large cardamom, fennel	Less garlic, asafetida	Holy basil, curry leaves, mint
Pulses	In moderation, avoid Bengal gram	Avoid horse-gram and flat beans	Mostly good
Dry fruits	Very little	In moderation	Less
Sweets	Fine	Deserts from sugarcane juice, jiggery	Honey is advised
Fats	Oil, ghee, butter	Ghee. mustard, gingelly oil less.	Less
Diet to avoid	Dry and cold foods, carbonated drinks, unripe fruit	Hot, spicy foods and wines	Cold, creamy foods, deserts, carbonated & frozen foods
Diet intake pattern	Eat small meals but frequently.	Sustain normal blood sugar, eat regularly	Maintain proper gaps for slow digestion

Sheet 2

Favorable Lifestyle Chart

Lifestyle	Vata Type	Pitta Type	Kapha Type
Sleep pattern	Sleep pattern needs to organized and followed.	Avoid lights at bedtime, sleep more relaxed	Day sleep is strictly forbidden
Exercise & Yoga	Follow routine. *Bhastrika, kapalbhati* and alternate deep breathing helps.	*Sheetali* and *sheetkari pranayaams* are cooling. Deep breathing through left nostril.	All *prayanaams* vigorously. Deep breathing through right nostril.
Sex life	Desire & energy needs to be saved	Not too vigorous.	Moderate to good
Emotional support	Take up a gentle hobby to remain distracted of unnecessary apprehensions.	Spend time with friends who are not competition for you.	Be more talkative with friends where you can relieve and give vent to emotions.
Massage therapy	Needs to be followed religiously, warming oils are suitable	Compassionate massage with soothing and cooling oil, crème	Stimulating, deep tissue or dry massage
Aroma therapy	Lavender, saffron, cinnamon	Sandalwood, rose, jasmine	Basil, eucalyptus oils
Colour therapy	Green colour	Blue, violet, indigo	Yellow, red, orange

Panchkarma techniques	Vasti (Enemas)	Virechana (Purgation)	Vamana (vomiting)
Remedial diet	Oil	Ghee	Honey
Important message	Follow routine	De-stress occasionally	utilize the stored energy
Seasonal intervention	More care during Rainy season which vitiates Vata	Autumn vitiates pitta so needs more concern.	Spring vitiates kapha and needs more care.

The three friends handed over their work sheets to Dr Wizard. "Ok ladies, please give me 15 minutes to go through your Self Care—Diet and Lifestyle Recommendation Crux Sheets as you have mentioned in two or three sentences right after my instruction. This is your last exercise in my class and provides me the gist of your take on Dosha healing, the ancient science of Healing through Ayurveda and I want to read this right now and right here in front of your eyes," he announced.

The girls showed apparent signs of discomfort on hearing this, but Dr Ayur Wizard simply ignored them and went about reading their papers.

After about 10-15 minutes, which seemed like a lifetime to the three, he said, "Now, I have good news and bad news for you. I will tell you the bad news first. Actually, there is nothing bad or good, it is only about your basic reaction. Well, as far as my experience with the three of you, I have noticed that writing about and assessing your own selves is not a happy note for you. And I can tell you there are three different reasons for the similar reaction that you bring forth. Whereas Vani who is typically Vata type has been disturbed with apprehension, Pia the Pitta girl looks at this as needless evaluation and Kapha type individual that is Kavya, has generally found this tedious paper work rather interfering with her tranquil state. Am I wrong?" The girls shook their heads.

"The so-called 'Bad' news for you is that exactly after six months from today, all three of you have to write something for me. This time, you have to write a letter. It has to talk about your personal experiences good or bad, broadly in the arena of healing (physical and mental), relationships and life. And this should mention how Dosha Healing—the ancient science of Healing through Ayurveda—has helped you. These would not be simple letters inscribed on a piece of paper for me, but the most fruitful return gift or *'Guru Dakshina'* as they name it," he said.

This clearly stunned the girls. "Believe me, more than the fees that you pay to be a part of my class, these letters are my real reward!" he said, waving a thick bundle of letters (probably from his earlier participants) in front of them.

Kavya was a little more moved than her friends. Did she just detect a hint of wetness in Dr Wizard's eyes? 'I'm probably imagining things,' she said to herself.

His voice pulled her out of her reverie. "Now, for the good news! Since this is your last class with me, I wanted to treat you girls to some refreshments that are waiting for you outside in the garden. Please enjoy the refreshments and see me after fifteen minutes," with that he left.

lifestyle changes that are significant for you," said Dr Wizard, happily handing over the sheets to them. "You may take these exercise sheets with you and keep them for ready reference."

"Before we say our goodbyes, I want to share a story," he said and immediately there were murmurs in the class. "This is story from Panchtantra, the ancient Indian wisdom of stories with lessons. Long, long ago, three fish Anagatavidhata, Pratyutpannamati and Yadbhavishya lived with their families in a pond. Anagatavidhata had a practical approach and would plan her actions in advance. You can call her 'Plan Ahead'. Pratyutpannamati was quick in judgment as well as reaction. You can call her 'Think fast'. And the third fish Yadbhavishya, the youngest of them all, loved to relax and linger with deliberation. You may call her 'Wait and see'.

"One day, the three fish overheard a fisherman tell his friend about his plans to cast a net in the pond the next day. On hearing this, the three reacted. However, their reactions were distinctly different. The first fish, Anagatavidhata or Plan Ahead, took immediate decision and told her friends that she would swim down the river that very night to save herself. And that was what she did. The second fish, Pratyutpannamati or Think Fast, was sure that she would come up with a plan at the time of emergency and decided to stay back. While the third fish Yadbhavishya or Wait and See remained lethargic and relaxed telling herself that as she could not think about how to handle the situation immediately therefore it was better to wait and watch till the time arrives. The next day, when the fisherman cast his net, the first fish Plan Ahead had already escaped. But Think Fast and Wait and See were caught. Think Fast quickly rolled its belly up and pretended to be dead. This made the fisherman leave the fish and throw it back into the safety of the water. But, Wait and See ended up in the fish market.

"Now, my question to you is: Tell me the basic personality types of the three fishes in the story that I just narrated,"

All three friends spoke in chorus, "Plan ahead is Vata type, Think fast is a Pitta type and Wait and watch is Kapha type."

"Correct! My students are now really familiar with the concept of Dosha Healing. Good job!" he said, applauding them.

"Coming back to the story, though in the story, only the last fish is caught, but in real life, it could be any of the three. Always try to keep this in your minds. If the first fish which is Vata type was not balanced, the same Vata dosha which is providing her with alertness and velocity could make her rather anxious and unable to take the right decision. And this is how the fish could have lost the battle. Similarly, if the second one which is Pitta type fell out of kilter, she would have lost her basic instinct of being intelligent and courageous, and could become impatient or frustrated and thus would have given in to her own mental truce. On the other hand, the third fish which is Kapha type could save herself from all negative consequences, if she was in better balance with her basic Kapha dosha providing her with sturdy and meticulous approach to the situation," he said, looking at each one of them.

"Therefore friends, my final advice to you is this: You have a typical dosha that is different from each other's. And your innate dosha not only forms your basic structure, but also your mental temperament—your complete personality. You have both positives and negatives within you because of your particular dosha. Now, it is for you to decide which traits you are going to cash on and which ones to curtail to keep your innate dosha balanced. Keep the ball in your court form now onwards and take the lead as well as responsibility of your holistic wellbeing. And this is what Dosha healing—The ancient science of Healing through Ayurveda is all about. Keep in touch. And I'm looking forward to receiving those letters. All the best," he said, saying his final goodbyes.

And before he left he gave them his parting gifts in the form of additional sheets for them to take home. The sheets had 'More about Self Care' written on them.

Sheet

More about Self Care I

All the three vitiated or imbalanced doshas can be brought back to their original form. The principle that works in this regard is to bring about a change in the Aahara (diet pattern) and in the Vihara (everyday activities that make your lifestyle). It has been specifically acknowledged in Ayurveda texts that a dosha or body humour tends to get aggravated mainly by undertaking Aahara and Vihara of the properties similar to the respective Doshas. This is because 'like increases like'. Hence, the vitiated or aggravated Dosha can only be nullified by undertaking the diet regimen and activities which oppose that particular body humor or dosha in properties.

Ayurveda says that it is important to eat and live in accordance to your basic dosha, to have a balancing effect upon the dominant dosha or do things that will pacify and balance the dosha that has become excessive or aggravated. Ayurveda approach to restore the balance would be to make use of diet, medicine, therapy and lifestyle, all in contrasting properties of the aggravated humour to alleviate the same.

Self-Care for Vata Types

Ayurveda advises that to combat Vata imbalance, one needs to take charge of his diet and routine just like serving a close friend (sweet, oily and unctuous).

'Varatam snehanam mitravata'

Therefore, the Vata person needs to be make changes in diet and lifestyle slowly and steadily just like taking care of a potted plant.

When Vata has to be brought back into balance, it's of foremost priority to take up diet and routine that is in contrary to the traits of Vata dosha.

- Ruksha—dry, rough. The dryness of Vata needs to be countered with use of oil both internally as well as externally. Whole body massage with some previously warmed oil or with oil having hot potency is advised like mustard oil, sesame seed oil. Also, the diet that is warm, heavy and unctuous is recommended for Vata types.

- Laghu—light. In contrast to this property of the air, diet needs to be somewhat heavy in nature and the stomach needs to refilled more frequently with nourishing food. Food that is high in nutritive value and energy giving helps subside the imbalanced Vata dosha.

- Shita—cold, cooling. To counter this, warm and freshly cooked foods with hot potency are recommended. Ayurveda also suggests using hot bandages on body parts and warm poultice especially in cold climatic conditions. Indulging in activities like oiling of the body and steam, sauna, hot fomentation, sun bath, pressing or kneading body parts with warm hands, hot tub bath and sprinkling of hot water onto the body parts (especially Vata specific area below the umbilicus) helps subside the effects of the dosha.

- Sukshma—subtle, penetrating. Relaxing attitude, regulating the sleep pattern and following stability in work and environment is needed. Meditation and yoga breathing techniques need to be followed daily. This also helps to keep the mind quiet, as energy needs to be conserved. Relaxing both body and mind from time to time is to be made an eminent practice.

- Khara—raw, loose. Unyielding daily schedules and managing timetables are desirable. Maintaining silent and concentration periods help. Taking a nap or resting in a favourable environment without any stimuli too helps. Also, as the mental state of *Rajas Guna* is pre-dominant in Vata dosha, the Vata type individuals need to focus more on the positive mental traits of creativeness, zest and flexibility. Herbs like *Brahmi* and *Shankhpushpi,* which are natural brain tonics and supportive to central nervous system are recommended.

- Vishada—clear, transparent. Contrary to this trait, avoiding of undue stress and physical exertion and also taking in of warm thick vegetable soups with Vata pacifying condiments is to be practiced. Stimulating and digestive herb and condiment powders are needed for keeping the gastric fire invigorated. This is because Ayurveda states that the Vata types naturally have disturbed gastric fire or *vishamagni.*

While considering diet for Vata types, as Vata is naturally erratic, rough and light, to balance these properties the diet of a Vata type person needs to be warm, heavy and unctuous. Ayurveda recommends the three basic tastes in everyday diet for Vata types viz. sweet, salty and sour and yet the other three tastes i.e. pungent, bitter and astringent need to be restricted in diet.

Therapeutically, when Vata is highly imbalanced and giving rise to the 80 types of Vata ailments, Ayurveda recommends vasti, which is a variety of Panchkarma therapy. *Vastivartaharana shreshtam* (CS Su 25/39)

According to Ayurveda text, most activities and diet recommended for the winter season would benefit a Vata type of individual. Thus, while narrating the regime for the winter season; the Ayurveda text has rightly advocated the ahara (diet pattern) and vihara (daily activities) of a Vata individual.

Self Care for Pitta type

According to Ayurveda text, one has to treat Pitta as one would treat a son-in-law (especially in India)—with paramount care and compassion, serving him sweetened cold drinks and comforting foods.

'*Pitam jamatramiva madhur sheetalayajayate*'

To combat Pitta imbalance, Ayurveda recommends taking up a regime that renders opposing qualities as that of the Pitta dosha or the fire body humour.

- Ushana—hot. Going against this characteristic, cool and calming foods and cold drinks prove to be relieving. It is also suggested that a Pitta type individual spends most of his time in a colder environment. Cold tub bath and using soft, cooling, fragrant herbs like sandalwood, camphor, khas khas and rose in the form of body pastes is beneficial. Also activities like bathing and swimming in cool and fragrant water would be soothing for balancing Pitta.

- Tikshana—sharp. Maintaining an easy-going attitude and evading potent and intense foods is needed. As the gastric fire is vigorous, digestion in Pitta types is generally upright. Therefore, a Pitta person needs to snack often (to avoid gastric burning and hypoglycemia). Also, possessing virtues of a sharp intellect and memory may at times hamper the mental balance and aggravate Pitta. Therefore, the Pitta individual needs to incorporate necessary periodic holidays and also take up an easy hobby.

- Drava—flowing, fluid. All stressful conditions and nervous pressures need to be avoided. Subtle meditation and Bhramari pranayaam is advised. Also, the breathing exercises need to be commenced with left nostril, as this leaves an overall cooling effect. Whenever indulging in exercise, it needs to be practiced moderately or until self-challenging situations arise. As for physical and mental relaxation, Ayurveda suggests that Pitta individual may include ornaments as necklaces of fragrant sandalwood, lotus or pearls and listen to soft melodies.

- Sara—mobile. Mobility needs to be hampered occasionally and physical and mental rest is much needed for Pitta types. For thoughtful Pitta relaxation and sleep and to calm the strangled nerves, the room needs to be kept rightly dark and mildly scented with rose petals, lavender oil drops or henna leaves. Ayurveda also suggests taking a nap in the moonlight or amidst cool air and showers, or in cool dark shade. Rejoicing and relaxing in scenery splendor would surely have a serene effect on the mind.

- Snigdha—oily, viscous. As you already have more of fire in your system, fried and unctuous diet needs to be restricted. Also any application of oils on body may be replaced by soothing crèmes. As for massage, choice of oil should be cooling one like coconut, or even better fragrant and soothing and calming crèmes. Massage with ghee is recommended.

The mental state of Satwa Guna is predominant in Pitta. This virtue may be easily maintained by the Pitta type by incorporating mental positive traits of being logical, decisive and ambitious.

Mainly while deciding the Pitta diet, as the quality of Pitta is heat, there is easy combustion of food, which would further results into low levels of blood sugar. Therefore, snacking is allowed with sweets, succulent fruits, sweetened deserts and fruit juices. Also, the three tastes that are mainly recommended for Pitta balance are sweet, bitter and astringent. The other three tastes i.e. pungent, sour and salty need to be restricted. Ghee (clarified butter) is good especially the ghee prepared with cooling and calming herbs. Milk and milk products are also optional for Pitta types.

Pitta aggravation may lead to 40 types of diseases. Ayurveda counsels Panchkarma treatment with virechan karma or inducting purgatives and this is considered to be the best possible therapy for subsiding and imbalanced fire humor. The therapy of Virechana (inducing purgation) and use of ghee and also milk both externally and internally has been suggested so as to calm the exacerbated Pitta.

Pitta lifestyle and diet is analogous to the ones advocated in summers. Or in summers we should lead a life like a Pitta person.

Self care for Kapha Type

Ayurveda suggests that a Kapha type individual could do himself good only if he treats himself just like he would treat his enemy.

'*Kapham durjanava tikshanaya*'

Kapha imbalance may be corrected by the Kapha types being tough and strict with themselves. This is because the stubborn Kapha is rather tricky to treat because of the inert trait of the earth element that this dosha imbibes. Hence, all intricate activities as well as potent and stimulating diet are meant for the Kapha types.

- Guru—heavy. Kapha types need to avoid overeating, nibbling on heavy foods and rather they need to eat an intense and potent diet. Most of the stimulating spices and condiments are good for them. They also need to engage in all sorts of physical work, to use up all that stored energy. Ayurveda recommends activities like long walks, running and exercise, participation in strenuous games like aerobics and swimming, avoiding sleeping during the day and keeping awake till late hours, taking up wrestling and bodily fights.

- Snigdha—oily, viscous. A diet heavy in fried and oily foods is not recommended. They also need to avoid emollient and grease—even the external application of oils on the body has to be discouraged. They can opt for dry massages that are deep tissue and stimulating using rough and coarse powder. Also, gargles with pungent substances, use of rough bedclothes and overall living in dry environment is good for them.

- Pichhila—turbid, gelatinous. Intake of thick and slimy foods needs to be restricted. Using the stored energy in any and every form, even by talking more, is recommended. As for mental support, meditation is also a necessity for Kapha person inculcating erect posture and using fragrant and stimulating aromas.

- Shita—cold, cooling. They can offset cold climes by moving on to warmer surroundings and having a warm diet. To combat the property of cold, Ayurveda suggests some typical diet and lifestyle measures: sun bathing, hot tub bath, steam inhalation (Kapha resides more in and above the chest), applying hot fomentation and poultice made from potent herbs like ajwain and saunth (dried ginger powder) over the forehead. Ayurveda also recommends hot steam bath, using of intense nasal errhines (nasya) and gargles. Even the water used for drinking should be preferably warm to hot, with potent herbs and condiments boiled in it.

- Sthula—coarse. Eating a light diet and periodical fasting is beneficial for the Kapha types. It needs to be understood that as empty stomach aids digestion, it is therefore suggested that a Kapha type individual maintains steady intervals between two meals. Waking up early also helps. Kapha dosha is naturally on the rise during the morning time (6 to 10am) and therefore being more active during this time of the day is needed.

- Sthira—stable, motionless. Kapha types need to keep on the move both physically as well as mentally. Taking up manual undertakings is beneficial. Kapha digestion is generally slow and yet fairly sound, therefore due to slow digestion, the Kapha type needs to avoid snacking between meals. Ayurveda advocates Kapha types to undertake optimal exercise and yoga, long brisk walks, Pranayamas, hard sports like swimming, jogging, cycling, climbing that would help to use up needlessly conserved energy.

- Slakshma—smooth. Using coarse cloth textures and more often taking up of strenuous tasks spontaneously and voluntarily proves beneficial.

The mental state of Tamas Guna naturally dominates Kapha. Therefore, consciously integrating positive emotions of harmony, empathy and caring is needed.

Diet management for the Kapha types counsels including the three rasas (tastes) viz. pungent, bitter and astringent in the meals while keeping sweet, salty and sour to the minimum. Stimulation and warmth are the two indispensable credentials for balancing the Kapha dosha.

Ayurveda states that Kapha aggravation and imbalance may result in 20 types of ailments. As for Panchkarma therapy, Vamana or inducing forceful vomiting is the best possible way to extract the phlegm stuck in the stomach, chest and throat region.

To balance Kapha, the ancient text has approved following a regimen and daily routine required to be inculcated during the Spring season.

More about self care II

Basics of Dosha Healing

- You must know and understand your basic dosha type

- Try to keep your basic *dosha* in its natural harmony.

- Watch out for any variation or aggravation in your basic dosha.

- Be prepared to incorporate everyday diet and lifestyle modifications according to your dosha type or *Prakriti*.

SELF CARE TIPS FOR VATA TYPE

- Bring slow and steady changes.

- Adequate sleep is a must with proper sleep pattern.

- Schedule and regularize your everyday activities.

- Get massages.

- Halt purposefully at times and practice relaxation techniques.

- Eat in moderation but more frequently to support your digestion.

- Practice Yoga with patience and controlled movements.

- Conserve your energy whenever possible.

- Take occasional vocal and mental rest, practice solitary meditation or engage in a leisure activity.

- Write your daily plans and stick to it.

- Ease your mind and calm your tensed nerves more often. Practice will help.

- Stop jumping to creative ideas and losing patience. Teaming up with *Kapha* and *Pitta* types and working together with other dosha types will help.

SELF CARE TIPS FOR PITTA TYPE

- Treat yourself more tenderly and less logically.

- Sleep in a dark environment as it makes you less sensitive to disrupted patterns of mind.

- Take a light massage once in a while with soothing crèmes to help relax.

- Relax and associate more with likeminded people.

- Take up hobbies like painting, gardening just for the sake of relaxation and enjoyment and not for competition.

- Take out time for meditation and rejuvenation.

- Snack frequently on sweet fruits and nuts because you have a voracious digestive fire.

- Get moderate exercise in colder environment.

- Try being less judgmental, less ambitious and less coordinated occasionally.

SELF CARE TIPS FOR KAPHA TYPE

- Be strict and pushy with yourself.

- Get up early and avoid daytime naps.

- Try making your life less relaxed both physically and mentally.

- Take dry massages or stimulating, deep tissue massages.

- Eat light and avoid snacking.

- Avoid overeating and as a compensation of affection.

- Make more friends who are enthusiastic and supportive. Though a good listener, take up sessions of long walks with friends and agreeable companions.

- Take up exercises like climbing, walking, gardening with company that keeps you going.

- Bring drastic but minor changes in lifestyle and stick to them.

- Meditate early morning or in the evening. Use some incense and sit upright.

THE FINAL VERDICT

- For Vata Type: **BE ORGANIZED AND KEEP CONTROL**

- For Pitta Type: **TAKE IT EASY AND KEEP THE COOL**

- For Kapha Type: **USE YOUR ENERGY AND KEEP MOTIVATED**.

EPILOGUE

CHAPTER 16

Six months later . . .

Vani's letter to Dr Wizard

Vani had been waiting to write back to Dr Ayur Wizard. Strangely, she could never see herself patiently looking forward to some event so much uncomplainingly and with such zeal and enthusiasm. She felt like a champ and why not? She had won a battle with herself, if not with the entire world. Here's what she wrote . . .

Dear Dr Wizard,

Since I returned from Delhi six months back, I have pinned up my Self-Care sheet on the mirror because I'm in the habit of peeping into the mirror many times a day. There are several areas of my triumph. First and foremost is my health. I now feel healthy, much healthy. My skin is behaving right after all these years, and I am actually sleeping through the nights.

Little matters that used to scream for my attention seem to go un-noticed. And that's really good. More than Dosha healing, perhaps it's the meditation that has helped me in this regard. I'm listing my personal achievements in areas of heath, wisdom, relationships and career.

Health: As I mentioned earlier, my skin maladies are almost gone and there is less dryness. My skin feels supple and glowing many a times and my hair is now manageable, thanks to the regular oil massages. In addition, my digestion problems too have reduced and my constipation is on its way out. I sleep throughout the night and welcome even the day-time naps. I have to admit that I now feel more energetic and balanced.

Wisdom: On this score too, I am doing well and now I have fewer apprehensions, more patience and confidence. I am able to analyse before reacting on impulse. I almost feel like a new person, one who is more independent than before. I am able to handle important matters in life, and at the same time ignore pointless things. My biggest achievement though is that I am now able to steer clear of my former mentally anxious state.

Relationships: Harshit, my hubby, has shown more persistence towards me and surprisingly I tend to receive his philosophies with patience. My daughter is doing well and listening to me, though it still could be the other way round. But we're more like friends now.

Lifestyle: You'd be pleased to know that I have incorporated most of the healing modalities that you have recommended like daily yoga, meditation, necessary massage and oiling of my body; following the right diet and overall regularising my routine. I must say that all this has given me a new level of fitness, enthusiasm and self-control. My gratitude!

Career: My relationship with my boss has improved drastically. I am able to handle the workload efficiently and have noticed that I have somehow become more creative. Actually, I am now an overall responsible person and I think it has also helped me to get a salary hike. For this accomplishment, the credit goes straight to you.

Sincerely yours,
Vani

Pia's letter to Dr Wizard

Pia's letter to Ayur wizard was neatly done and as was expected was to the point, literally. She had listed 10 points, summarising her success story in them.

Hello Dr Ayur Wizard,

I'm sure you have been waiting to hear back from us. I am happy to tell you that despite my initial reservations, I have experienced a positive transformation. I am listing the changes below:

1. My hyperacidity is gone. So are the migraine headaches, though they are not completely gone but have reduced both in frequency and severity. Also, my blood pressure is normalising and it seems that my dependency on hypertension medicines would decline soon.

2. About my actions and reactions, the world is still crazy as hell. They will never improve. But now, I try to curtail my impulse to react and this actually gives me some peace.

3. My sleep pattern has been better. I avoid late nights and am rather comfortable with my own enforced nap during the day-time. And I must agree that this has helped keep my stress levels down.

4. Ever since my diet has been altered, it has helped in relieving the occasional weakness

and drained-out state. One tip that has worked out well with me is that I still feel hungrier than others at home, yet I generally take some sweet and cold food stuff, before my energy is completely drained.

5. In everyday lifestyle, I have included swimming as a daily activity, and I think it has proved to be a blessing for my health.

6. I have noticed this change in my attitude (not sure how long it's going to last). However, even though there are irrational people around me, I can be patient, calm and somehow detached. This virtue has not come suddenly to me. I started with this practice first at home, and then at my job and the outside world.

7. I'm much choosy about not only my own tastes, but also the tastes of entire family. They have had sermons from me in this regard many times now, but I'm sure they agree. As far as my diet is concerned, sweet is part of my everyday tastes, although indulging in the bitter and astringent foods is not at all easy for me. But health is a priority always. Therefore, Karela juice is also acceptable once in a while.

8. I do remain busy as it is a part and parcel of metropolitan lifestyle. But yes, taking leisure breaks from my tight schedules help me rejuvenate. And I want to thank you for this, Dr Wizard. Earlier I guess I would always feel

my brow is frowning and tensed up, but now off-and-on with practice, I can make myself smile.

9. I am also learning to maintain my physical cool as much I'm doing it for my mind. Though, following a liquid diet, having fruit juices, cooling herbs and ghee as you had recommended is comparatively easier than maintaining the mental cool. But I have noted down all the points clearly in my dairy and tend to refer to them as and when I feel 'heated-up' The best part is . . . this simple bodily reaction warns me immediately of my dosha imbalance setting in.

10. Lastly, I want to thank you personally. I do not feel reluctant to disclose that when I was in your class I was sort of mystified and confounded with all the stuff about dosha healing that you would preach to us. Of course, I wanted to try it all. It has worked out well for me and is much better than stuffing myself with all those medications. I also want to tell you that now I plan to take this knowledge about dosha healing to a wider audience in this country and abroad as well. Be ready Dr Ayur Wizard, soon you will be inundated with invitations for talks and workshops on dosha healing. Of course, you can rely on me for supporting you whole heartedly in the same.

Best Regards,
Pia

Kavya's letter to Dr Ayur Wizard

Hello Dr Ayur wizard,

It gives me great pleasure as well as comfort to write to you. The 'Dosha healing' sessions that I have taken under your expert guidance have completely transformed my world, for the better.

I am starting my letter with good news for you. Actually, this is an emotion to be hidden from the entire world, but I know this well and good that you will understand. You know Dr Ayur wizard, I'm pregnant. In the next year, with God's grace we will be blessed with a baby of our own. And please do not worry. This has not interfered with my love for my daughters at all. Rather, this goodness had filled me with gratitude— towards you, the ancient science of dosha healing as well as towards my two sweet little girls.

I believe that somewhere, it is due to their goodwill and prayers that I got this opportunity of my lifetime to meet you in person and understand the relevance and role of the 5,000-year-old science of Ayurveda in our lives. The second good news is I have lost more than 10 pounds. Actually, within me I knew that my obesity and childlessness are inter-related. Kindly accept my heartfelt gratitude for helping me break the vicious cycle once and for all with the potent tool of dosha healing.

Not only this, my sinus headaches and nasal congestion are much better in just six months. I have been very strict and much pushy with myself. But I have taken this as biggest lesson from you. You helped me understand that this was my weak point and let me tell you that this is where I have always lost the battle even before fighting it. Although, I must tell you that this was not at all easy for me. Rather, for the first month, it was hard as hell. You know, my husband would pity me and tell me to take it easy. He would say that it was just a class and if I was finding it so difficult to follow, then I could just leave it and forget about it. But I had made up my mind and was totally sold on what you taught me. Then, as I continued consciously taking control of my diet as well as lifestyle, I could sense improvement steadily coming into my physical health, which further propelled my mental state. I had begun to lose the flab and felt light and somewhat balanced. After three months, I had mostly trained my mind. You will be surprised to know, I'm not a foodie anymore. I really do not know how I could overcome it. Again, I guess it's all about the repeated emphasis you had placed on being stringent for balancing the Kapha dosha. I have almost exterminated my taste buds with the unpleasant tastes. I even go out in fresh air for brisk walk (even if it has to be four times a day) every time I sense myself going weak on my commitment or getting lethargic.

Along with all this, I am now much at ease with my husband. Can't say why, but this is another positive change I have noticed lately. I trust him more and am not so possessive about him. This has surely improved our relationship. I'm sure the subtle meditation that you had suggested has categorically worked in this arena.

With much gratitude, love and blessed wishes for you and for the concept of Dosha Healing—The Ancient wisdom of Healing through Ayurveda!

Your student,

Kavya ☺

....

REFERENCES

Krishan Sonica.2011.Healing through Ayurveda—Tips for Dosha Understanding and Self Care. Rupa Publication India Pvt Ltd.

Charaka Sanhita of Agnivesh by Vaidya Sri Satya Narayan Shastri

Glossary

- Ayurveda—The age old science of life and longevity.

- Aakasha—Denotes ether or the sky and is one of five basic natural elements that make up the entire natural existence.

- Vayu—Denotes the air which is one of five basic natural elements that make up the entire natural existence.

- Tejas—Denotes fire and is one of five basic natural elements that make up the entire natural existence.

- Jala—Denotes water and is one of five basic natural elements that make up the entire natural existence.

- Prithvi—Denotes the earth and is one of five basic natural elements that make up the entire natural existence.

- Panchbhoota—The five natural basic elements or the fundamental building blocks viz. ether, air, fire, water and earth.

- Dosha—The three body humors or the bio-regulatory principles of the body.

- Vata—Air body humor that is the product of ether and air and manifests as moving bio-regulatory principle in human body.

- Pitta—Fire humor of the body which attributes to process of physiological activities of metabolism, assimilation, digestion etc in the body.

- Kapha—Phlegm body humor which is the bio-regulatory principle that sources formation, nutrition and sustenance of the physical body.

- Humor—The three bio-regulatory principles viz. air; fire and phlegm in the body as recognized by Ayurveda.

- Ruksha—dry

- Laghu—light

- Shita—cold or cool

- Sukshma—minute

- Khara—rough

- Vishada—transparent or clear

- Guna—Basic trait or the natural attribute

- Ushana—hot

- Tikshana—sharp

- Drava—liquid

- Sara—fluid

- Snigdha—oily, unctuous

- Satwa Guna—Positive and balanced mental state.

- Rajas Guna—Variable and erratic mental attribute.

- Tamas Guna—Negative and depressed state of the mind.

- Prakriti—The natural bodily constitution and mental temperament of an individual.

- Satwa—Natural essence

- Guru—heavy

- Pichhila—Slimy or greasy

- Sthula—heavy, gross

- Sthira—Static

- Slakshma—Smooth

- Aahara—Diet

- Vihara—Everyday lifestyle

- Vishamagni—Disrupted gastric fire.

- Panchkarma—The prime five cleansing processes of the body viz. inducing vomiting, purgation, the enemas and nasal errhines.

- Mahabhootas—Basic elements

- Dhatus—Body tissues

- Tridosha—The three body humors viz. air, fire and phlegm.

- Vasti—Enema

- Virechana—Purgation

- Vamana—Vomiting

- Satvic—Relating to positive mental state.

- Shloka—Ancient Sanskrit adage.

ENDORSEMENTS

"How refreshing to learn through a binding and riveting story. As always, Dr. Sonica has a way of keeping you spellbound while she imparts incredibly wise and meaningful lessons about the ancient wisdom of Ayurveda. Will it change your life? Read this inspiring story and find out how your life can improve."

Anton Van Den Berg

Motivator, Speaker, Business Executive, Developer of People, Gauteng, South Africa.

"Dr Sonica Krishan manages to bring to life in her pages the bond of friendship, the trials of life's heart wrenching challenges, and weaves in seamlessly

Ayurveda health and healing in a non-threatening, easy to understand way."

Carly Alyssa Thorne

Speaker, Author, ~ Co-Author of "Contemplating Change, One's Quotes with Paul Smith, Agoura Hills, California.

"Dr. Sonica is a wonderful storyteller who, in this book, weaves the ancient wisdom of Ayurvedic Dosha healing with a beautiful tale of three childhood friends, reunited and whose lives are changed forever. You will be transformed by the wisdom as you read!"

Catherine Fenske

PhD (candidate), Spiritual Teacher, Reiki Master & Author of weekly column, "Joy To You" in the GJ Free Press, Colorado, USA.

"Dr. Sonica weaves the ancient wisdom of Ayurvedic Dosha healing throughout her beautiful tale of how the reuniting of three childhood friends changed their lives forever. A captivating read that will transform your own life!"

Debbie Friend

Master of Science in Exercise Physiology and Cardiac Rehabilitation. Certified Laughter Yoga Leader, Owner: Life Currents, Chicago, USA.

"Vital health facts presented in a catchy way. Human brain is wired for story, and the health facts are likely to stay in your sub-conscious mind and likely to contribute to your healthy habits and a preventive healthcare mind-set. The best part is all the information comes from the Ayurveda Queen herself!"

Dr Amit Nagpal

Dr Amit Nagpal is Author, Speaker & Coach in the area of inspirational & brand storytelling, New Delhi, India.

"Congratulations to Sonica Krishan for writing an easily accessible, entertaining and a truly unique book to introduce the reader to Ayurveda. Through creative storytelling, she has done an excellent job of explaining the three doshas, their effects on our lives and how the knowledge of Ayurveda can help us to find balance and health in our lives. May the lives of all who read this book be healed."

Dr. Marc Halpern

Author of Healing Your Life; Lessons on the Path of Ayurveda and President of the California College of Ayurveda, Nevada City, California.

"An introduction to Ayurveda, through a fictional story makes the reader hooked to read on. Dr Sonica

Krishan has for the first time made it easier to read and remember basics of Ayurveda."

Dr Talavane Krishna

MD, Founder, Indus Valley Ayurvedic Centre, Mysore, India

"When confronted with past betrayals by self and others, we can find the strength to soar beyond self-imposed limitations and successfully learn along the way to give love. Dr Sonica Krishan's book is going to be great help for you to learn just the same."

Jane Scarratt

Spiritual Kinesiologist, Gold Coast Australia.

"Sonica is an expert storyteller and health professional. Combine these traits and you have a brilliant novel that will hold you from beginning to end."

Linda Lycett

Dip Professional Editing, Spinner, Design Knitter and Publisher, Aurora House, Sydney, Australia.

"Healthy Living through Dosha Healing by Dr. Sonica Krishan is by far one of the best books ever written on the subject in my personal opinion! You will never have to buy another book on the subject.

Philippe Shock Matthews

Host: The Philippe Matthews Show - www.thepmshow.tv | Executive Director: The How Movement - www.howmovement. org | Amazon Bestselling Author: www.booksbypm.com

"Through story-telling, Dr. Krishan has brilliantly brought to life the modern day application and wisdom of the 5,000-year-old system of Dosha Healing in this new book. Using the intimacy and emotional depth allowed by fiction, she introduces us to the lives and loves of three women, effectively teaching us how Ayurveda's principles are just as applicable today to achieving balance and reaching our full human potential."

Rory Kelly Connor

Provocateur, Founder of the Official SexyPeeps™, Change Agent, Strategist, Certified Coach, Greater New York, USA.

"An amazing story about life but most importantly, about how we can all heal ourselves. In the most remarkable way, Dr. Sonica brings the ancient wisdom of Ayurveda in a way that our fast-paced minds can easily understand. Isn't that what the truth you're looking for is all about. I recommend this amazing story to anyone who wants to live happily ever after."

Roxana Jones

Best-selling author and energy healer dedicated to unify and heal the world through words, Los Angeles, California.

"This book creatively weaves together an ancient wisdom with an unfolding of self-discovery and friendship. It authentically invites readers not only to partake in a story resembling 'the search' of our time, to tap into the healing possibility of a dynamic science that could change lives forever."

Tanya Markul

Co-Founder & Editor of RebelleSociety.com, Copenhagen, Denmark.